# HEROES
# SAINTS
# AND YOGIS

## AND PEOPLE LIKE
## YOU AND ME

Tales of Self–Discovery and the Path of Sikh Dharma

Compiled by

MSS SHAKTI PARWHA KAUR KHALSA
and
MSS GURUKA SINGH KHALSA

and SS SAT MANDER KAUR KHALSA

Published by the Kundalini Research Institute
Training • Publishing • Research • Resources
PO Box 1819
Santa Cruz, NM 87567

www.kundaliniresearchinstitute.org

ISBN 978-1-934532-76-8

The editors are truly grateful to everyone who contributed articles to this collection and generously shared their personal stories. Thank you each and all!

Gurukirn Kaur for her article, "Celestial Communication"; Guru Rattan Kaur for her article about Miri Piri Academy; Livtar Singh for his piece on composing "The Song of the Khalsa"; Sadasat Singh for his adventure, "Destined to Stay"; Harjinder Ruby Kaur Khalsa for "Born in India & Raised in North America"; Dr. Sat-Kaur for her piece on the Sikh Dharma Ministry, and Sat Daya Singh for telling his personal journey.

Articles regarding Sikh Dharma are reprinted with permission from www.sikhdharma.org.

The Anand Sahib Translation on pages 159-161 is reprinted with permission from the author. Copyright 2008 by Ek Ong Kaar Kaur Khalsa. www.facebook.com/ekongkaarkhalsa. ekongkaar.blogspot.com

Editor & Creative Director: Sat Purkh Kaur Khalsa
Copy Editor: Sahib-Amar Kaur Khalsa
Cover Photo: Gurumustuk Singh Khalsa
Cover Design and Layout: Prana Projects: Ditta Khalsa, Biljana Spasovska
Photos by Gurumustuk Singh Khalsa. Used with permission.
Photo of Bhai Sahib Dyal Singh on page 139 by Satkirin Kaur Khalsa. Used with Permission.
Photo of Yogi Bhajan on page 21: (c) 1972 The Yogi Bhajan Photo Archive. Used with Permission. For more information see: www.yogibhajan.com/Photos.htm

# Table of Contents

····································

"When we say Sikh Dharma, we mean 'the path of the student.' Some people think it means a religion. Sikh means a student on a pathway to one's own Self: *from my head to my heart*. As a Sikh, the life of a person is fulfilled and enlightened, living as a householder[1] and a yogi."

— *Yogi Bhajan, July 12, 2001*

---

[1]  A person who lives in the everyday world, works, has a family, goes to school, etc.

# Dedication

*In Loving Memory*

☬

*Siri Singh Sahib,*

*Bhai Sahib, Harbhajan Singh Khalsa Yogiji*

*(Yogi Bhajan)*

*Who brought Sikh Dharma to life*

*in the Western Hemisphere.*

# Plane Talk

Inspiration for this poem came shortly after 9/11. My clothing attracted the interest of a man sitting across the aisle from me on an airplane. He asked me why I dressed the way I do, and a conversation ensued. Later, I wrote the following poem about our encounter.

— MSS Shakti Parwha Kaur Khalsa

Across the aisle, the lady with the smile

Is wearing, my goodness, a Turban!

Dressed all in white, a dazzling sight

Reading the newspaper, she seems quite urban.


My curiosity piqued, I cannot resist

Asking as politely as I can,

"Dear lady, what is the reason for your attire?

Please enlighten me; I'm just a simple man."

"Of course," she says, "I'm happy to comply

And explain the reasons, the wherefore, and the why

Of what we Sikhs call our bana, the distinctive dress

That makes us stand out – and might cause you some stress.


"You see, in our history, one of our leaders died for another religion's plight.

Sadly, many of his followers, when they saw him beheaded, ran away in fright.

His thirteen-year-old son, Gobind Rai, witnessed this shame,

Vowed that later in life, when Guru he became,

He'd ensure his Sikhs would have courage to stand up and be seen —

So he gave them a special uniform — with five symbols to wear.

Here's what these symbols mean:


"Turban is the crown of spirituality, it covers the gift of Kesh, long hair.

(We never cut it, because obviously, God wants it to grow there!)

The steel bracelet we wear is called a Kara, it says, "To God we belong."

(As Sikhs, we express our devotion through song.)


"A wooden comb in the hair, for cleanliness and care,

Tucked under the turban, can you see my Kanga there?

Katcheras – an underwear (take my word for it, I won't make a display)

Is worn to remind us to honor God's creative energy in every way.


Guru Nanak, whose students were called "sishyas" or Sikhs,

Was very adamant in his teaching:

'There is One God who breathes in all.'
So there's no need for us to go out preaching.

"When people ask about our Bana I tell them, 'Sikhs do not proselytize,'
But our clothing definitely does advertise —
Encouraging you to ask questions, then we can reply.'

"We respect all religions, races, genders, and colors; here's why:
God created each of us; the Truth of our identity, both yours and mine
Is that we are here on Earth for a human experience,
In essence we are beings born in Divine!
I know that's hard to accept, when you look at the surface,
And observe imperfections that seem so great,
But physical appearance, mental and emotional differences are just temporary
conveniences we use to function in this earthly state.

"Sikhs worship the word of God; the Shabd Guru is our guide.
A compilation of wisdom spoken by enlightened beings
Who experienced God deeply inside.

"Sikh tenets are simple, universal, and kind:
Get up early in the morning; clean your body and your mind,
Praise God's Name, then go to work and righteously earn
So you can share with those less fortunate, thus you will learn
'Tis more blessed to give than to receive,'
(When you try it, then you'll believe!)."

The lady with the smile continued, and I eagerly listened for more,
"Don't take my word for it," she said, "Doing is believing, that's really the core
Of the Sikh faith, for it's based on experience, and it's open to all.
Blessed are those who are inspired to respond to the call
To read from the Guru, to chant God's Name
You don't have to be a Sikh, just a seeker, to win life's game.

*"For, you see, it really is all God's Leelaa, His Divine play*
*In which we find ourselves on this particular day.*
*One Creator (Truth is His Name)*
*Created this creation in which we seek fortune and fame*
*But ultimately the purpose for which we were born*
*Is to discover SAT NAM, our own true identity,*
*and return to the lap of God from which we were torn."*

*"Oh, there's much more I could say, but I don't want to bore you."*
*I assured her I was truly sincere.*
*"Well then," she said, patting the place beside her,*
*"Why don't you come and sit over here?"*
*So I joined her, and for the rest of the flight,*
*I discovered what made her look so bright.*
*She told me about "Ang Sang Wahe Guru," affirming God's presence*
*in every part of your being.*
*Amazing faith, amazing grace, joyous commitment in her I was seeing!*

*"We are people of love, here to serve others*
*We recognize all people as sisters and brothers*
*Each life is sacred, God's precious gift to us*
*So we are pledged to defend it, if defend it we must.*
*We believe in kindness as the highest virtue, and it's peace we desire*
*But we are Soldier Saints when that's what's required.*

*"Faith in God and Guru gives us courage to face*
*Whatever happens through time and space.*
*We wish good to all, peace and love we do embrace*
*We pray for the protection of the whole human race."*

*The power and the beauty of love and duty, I saw in the lady in white*
*Her bana, her "ad," made me feel glad that destiny booked me on her flight.*

*So now when I see someone wearing a turban – perhaps even a bearded man,*
*I'll think, "He's a Sikh of the Guru," and strike up a conversation if I can.*

# Foreword

Sikh Dharma is a conscious way of living, a universal path that is open to anyone and everyone who wants to walk along it. Its principles and practices provide a blueprint for living a life of kindness, compassion, courage, and dignity. Living in peace and harmony with all people without discrimination, regardless of their gender, color, religious affiliation, political persuasion, status in life, caste, or creed is a fundamental principle of Sikh Dharma.

Legally, Sikh Dharma is a religion. Unfortunately, since the beginning of "civilization," religion has been used as an excuse for persecution, bigotry, and fanaticism. Even today, religions are being used to cause bloodshed, create animosity and perpetuate hatred among people, often as a front for gaining political or economic power. Yogi Bhajan came to the West to deliver a way of life, not a religion; so even though Sikh Dharma is a "religion," throughout this book we will present it as a path of consciousness, a *dharma*, a technology which delivers the human experience toward its own excellence and *cherdi kala*—ever-rising spirit.

Although Sikh Dharma is one of the youngest religions in the world, as well as being the fifth largest religion in the world, it is still relatively unknown in the West. One of the reasons there is so little known by the general public about Sikhs is that we don't try to convert anyone. Instead, we respect and defend everyone's right to worship God however they choose.

However, when the Twin Towers in New York were destroyed and 9/11 became a regular part of our vocabulary, anyone wearing a turban was immediately suspect. The need to explain the way we dress became glaringly apparent. Still I didn't really focus on this book until 2004, after a presentation for the Manhattan Beach Community Church in Southern California. After the slide show and Q&A, which was received with great interest, our gracious host, Dr. Louis Kilgore, asked if I could recommend three books that their Adult Discussion Group members could read to learn even more about the Sikhs. And with that question, I recognized how few resources were available for people to read and discover more about Sikh Dharma.

Of course, I told him about Macauliffe's six-volume treatise.[2] I had even brought my precious copy of *Sikh Dharma of the Western Hemisphere*[3] for show and tell. However, I didn't know of anything easily accessible—as well as reader friendly—currently on bookstore shelves that describes the *experience* of living as a Sikh. His request was the final catalyst that encouraged me to make this book happen.

There was a lot of material already available. What you hold in your hands is an edited collection of articles written by different people at different times, so the voice will change as well as the perspective, but we hope that it gives you a window into the lives of practicing Sikhs and the Teachings of Yogi Bhajan as they relate to Sikh Dharma and the path of consciousness.

I must confess, I still wish Sikh Dharma wasn't called a religion, because religions tend to separate people, which is contrary to the universal truth of Unity taught by Guru Nanak, the enlightened soul who became the first Sikh Guru. That being said, here it is, my humble attempt to share my understanding and especially my love for this way of life, a path I've been walking—in excellent company—for more than thirty-five years.

*MSS Shakti Parwha Kaur Khalsa*
*Los Angeles, California*
*2010*

---

[2] M. A. Macauliffe, *The Sikh Religion: Its Gurus, Sacred Writings and Authors*. Oxford Press, 1909 - ISBN 8175361328.
[3] Shanti Kaur Khalsa, *The History of Sikh Dharma of the Western Hemisphere*. Sikh Dharma Publications, 1995.

Chapter One

# Setting the Stage for the Aquarian Age

✖

Now that we have entered the 21st Century and are fast approaching the Aquarian Age, interfaith cooperation and communication is not only accepted but cultivated and sought out by so many people of faith. The Piscean walls of misunderstanding and fear are starting to crumble under the sheer weight of higher consciousness that is manifesting on this planet.

Many first generation Western Sikhs came to this path during the late sixties and early seventies in their search for expanded awareness and an experience of higher consciousness through their practice of yoga and meditation. We were "flower children" seeking the ideals of peace, cooperation and understanding. Sikh Dharma fit right in with that aspiration. In fact, the traditional Sikh prayer (*Ardas*), recited daily by Sikhs all over the world, ends with a phrase wishing "good to all!"[4]

# Becoming a Sikh in this Lifetime

Since 1974 when I officially declared my identity as a Sikh, I've always worn my turban in public. Strangers frequently ask me where I'm from. Probably they assume I'm from India. Depending upon the question and the questioner, I may simply answer, "I'm from Los Angeles," and keep moving. But if the person seems truly interested, then I add, "I'm a Sikh." If they look puzzled, I explain, "Sikh Dharma began in India, more than 500 years ago when Guru Nanak taught that there is One God who created all of this creation, and so there's no reason to fight about how to worship that One."

I say, "We wear distinctive clothing so that we are recognizable." I point at my turban and say, with a smile, "We don't proselytize, but we do advertise. We're vegetarians, we don't drink or smoke. We believe in honoring God by living as our Creator made us; in other words, we don't cut our hair—ever. We don't smoke or take drugs[4], and we honor the sanctity of marriage." And then I may add, "There are 25 million Sikhs throughout the world."

I wasn't born wearing a turban, and I was certainly never converted! It was simply that when I learned about the Sikh values and experienced the benefits of its practices, my soul recognized my identity as a Sikh and my heart welcomed it once again. A turban then became a permanent part of the way I dress (*bana*), which identifies me as a Sikh. Every time I tie those yards of cloth around my head, I am reminded of my commitment to live the Sikh way of life.

## Flashback

In 1966, when I was simply an American tourist visiting various holy shrines in India, a bearded gentleman wearing a turban approached me at the Mahatma Gandhi memorial in Delhi. He said, "I've noticed you several times at these places, and I'd like to tell you about the Sikh religion." I said, "Thank you very much, but I'm not interested." He politely withdrew and that was the end of that—at least I thought so at the time—until December of 1968 in Los Angeles, California, when I met another bearded gentleman wearing a turban. This Sikh was a yogi.

---

[4] Except as medically prescribed, of course!

# *Meeting Yogi Bhajan*

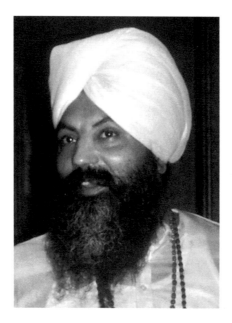

At the time, I was definitely not looking for a religion. In fact, I wasn't even looking for a teacher. When I first met Harbhajan Singh Puri, I had no idea that this man, who towered over everyone at 6' 2" and wore a pink turban, black velvet shoes that curled up at the toes, and white trousers with a thin black window-pane design, would soon become the world famous Yogi Bhajan, founder of 3HO Foundation, Master of Kundalini Yoga, spiritual teacher to hundreds of thousands, and eventually the Chief Religious and Administrative Authority for Sikhs in the Western Hemisphere with the unique ministerial title of "Siri Singh Sahib." If he had started preaching about religion, I would have run in the opposite direction. Instead, he told me that he had come to teach Kundalini Yoga. He was very specific: he was not here to gather students, but rather to train teachers—and that's just what he did.

I drove him to the classes we arranged. His first "job" was at the YMCA in Alhambra, California. Each student paid $1.50 and "the Yogi" got 75 cents. Attendance grew. It was not long before he was invited to teach in colleges, universities, health clubs, and spiritual centers throughout America, and eventually all over the world.

Between the exercises in his classes, he talked about the meaning and purpose of life. He explained the virtues that give human beings value and make life worthwhile. He talked about the technology of being human and explained the Sikh practices that served those same principles of consciousness, meditation, and elevation. We were inspired and enthralled by the fascinating tales he told of noble Sikh men and women whose lives adorn the pages of Sikh history. They came to life for us as he recounted their deeds. Tales of their courage, sacrifice, and honor spoke to our hearts and awakened our souls. Sometimes he would enthusiastically emphasize a point by quoting *Gurbani* (the language of the Gurus). He didn't bother to translate; he seemed to expect us to understand.

When Yogi Bhajan came to the West, it was the *dawning* of the Aquarian Age. A new consciousness was being born on Earth. We are now in the 21-year Cusp period (1991-2012; divided into three 7-year increments) leading up to the actual arrival of the Aquarian Age. Yogi Bhajan explained back in November of 1991 that this period of transition from the Piscean to the Aquarian Age would bring increasingly greater turmoil and upheaval to the planet. All around us we can see the Piscean walls of misunderstanding and fear starting to crumble under the sheer weight of higher consciousness that is manifesting on this planet. The old Piscean Age was dominated by machines and hierarchies. The new Aquarian Age is ruled by awareness, information, and energy.

Yogi Bhajan told us, "What worked before, won't work now." And, "Nothing can remain hidden." We are now seeing that manifested every day. People are waking up. For some this brings fear, and for some, joy. As the Aquarian Age comes closer, the contrast between those who live in fear and those who live in love becomes more obvious every day, for the two states are mutually exclusive. As I write this, we are now less than a thousand days away from the true beginning of the Age of Aquarius.

For over thirty-five years, Yogi Bhajan gave his life and energy to train teachers of Kundalini Yoga to share tools for the healing, inspiration, and personal awareness urgently needed by humanity in this critical time and space.

. . . . . . . . . . . . . . . . . . . . . . . . . . . . . . . . . . . . . . . . . . . . . . . . . . . . . . . . . . . . . . . . . . .

*"We do not need new choices. We are flooded with choices. We need an elevated capacity to make choices. We do not need more information. We need the wisdom to use all the information. We do not need another religion. We need the experience of a Dharma that creates the spiritual fitness to act believably on our beliefs. The Shabd Guru is a special kind of technology with a unique contribution to develop potentials and handle the problems of the new Age—the Aquarian Age. In the body it produces vitality; in the complex of the mind it awakens intelligence and develops wisdom and intuition; in the heart it establishes compassion; in each person's consciousness it builds the clarity to act with fearless integrity. The Aquarian Age demands personal experience and the capacity to act. The Shabd Guru is available to all. You need not search. You need to practice, experience, incorporate, and express."[5]*

. . . . . . . . . . . . . . . . . . . . . . . . . . . . . . . . . . . . . . . . . . . . . . . . . . . . . . . . . . . . . . . . . . .

The Aquarian Age[6] isn't just something that we started singing about in the sixties! It's an actual measurable time period. Here's one way to understand the astronomical ages in context with the Four Yugas mentioned in the Vedic Puranas.

Picture yourself inside a gigantic circular room. The walls are totally covered with a huge canvas hung from floor to ceiling. There is apparently no beginning and no end. On your left, the first panel you see is painted Gold. It is labeled "Sat Yug." It stretches 40 feet. Walking slowly in a clockwise direction you see it flowing seamlessly into the next panel, which extends 30 feet. It is Silver and is marked "Treta Yug." Then you see the next panel, marked "Duapar Yug," comprising 20 feet of shining Copper (or Bronze). It merges into the fourth panel, resembling the color of Steel. This one represents the *"Kali Yug,"* the Machine Age. It's only

---

5    Yogi Bhajan, *Basis, Use and Impact of the Quantum Technology of the Shabd Guru by Siri Singh Sahib Bhai Sahib Harbhajan Singh Khalsa Yogiji, Ph.D. compiled by Mukhia Singh Sahib Dr. Gurucharan Singh Khalsa, Ph.D. - April 1995*

6    *Time And Space: The Four Yugas And The Aquarian Age.* Reprinted with permission from the Aquarian Times Magazine article by Shakti Parwha Kaur Khalsa

10 feet long, and then you're back at the beginning of the first 40-foot panel. It's another Golden Age, "Sat Yug." The cycle is continuous.

You step closer and read the fine print describing each panel, and learn that the Golden Age, the *Sat Yug* or *"Age of Truth Fully Revealed,"* lasts 1,728,000 human years. This Age is characterized by unity in One God, people living in peace and harmony with God's will.

. . . . . . . . . . . . . . . . . . . . . . . . . . . . . . . . . . . . . . . . . . . . . . . . . . . . . . . . . . . . . . . . . . . . . . . . . . . . . . . . . .

*"Man was one with the Divine, and he realized the vibration which this Cosmic Energy created to make Prakriti (manifestation). People meditated on the Nam ONG (Creator—the vibration of the divine.*

*"In the Treta Yug, the Silver Age, one-fourth of the Truth was hidden. People began to feel separate from God. The being became weak and recited Sohang (I am You), and through this vibration acknowledged their identity with the Divine."*[7]

—*Yogi Bhajan*

. . . . . . . . . . . . . . . . . . . . . . . . . . . . . . . . . . . . . . . . . . . . . . . . . . . . . . . . . . . . . . . . . . . . . . . . . . . . . . . . . .

Using God's gift of free will, humans digressed further and further from God's will and lost even more awareness of their sacred identity. When we reached the Duapar Yug, Truth was only half visible. People worshipped God in the form of idols and images, and recited ONG NAMO NARAYANA.[8] Righteousness declined and people turned to various religions in order to have a relationship with God.

Now, in the year 2010, we are in the Kali Yug, where disorder, distress, disease, despair, conflict, and war dominate, and people have even said, "God is dead." In this Dark Age,[9] Truth has been three-fourths obscured. We have been in this Kali Yug for over 5,000 years, and there are still 426,889 years remaining!

Astrological ages are different from the Vedic Yugas. An astrological age is a time period in astrology that parallels major changes in the development of the human race. It roughly corresponds to the time taken for the vernal equinox to move through one of the twelve constellations of the zodiac. The Ages in astrology, however, do not correspond to the actual constellation boundaries where the vernal equinox may be occurring in a given time.

So, how does the *Aquarian Age* fit into all this? Look closely, and you will see, painted in the foreground of the huge span of the Kali Yug panel, a short, thin horizontal brush stroke divided into twelve sequential sections. These are the various *Astrological Ages*.

It takes over 2,100 years for our Solar system to travel through each one of the Signs or constellations. (Astronomically, the Sun moves through the zodiac in reverse order from the *Astrological* sequence with which we are more familiar.)

So far, humanity has recorded events in the Astronomical Taurean Age, which was the time of Adam; followed by the Arian Age when Abraham came into the picture; and just about when the Roman Empire rose to power, our Sun entered Pisces. It was in this Piscean Age that Jesus was born. All of this took place during the Kali Yug.

---

[7]   Yogi Bhajan, "Code Mantra Sheet," August 8, 1971.
[8]   Salutations to the Creator and to God in human form.
[9]   Not to be confused with the historic "Dark Ages."

The Age of Aquarius is foretold by Jesus in the Aquarian Gospel:[10] *"And then the man who bears the pitcher will walk forth across an arc of heaven; the sign and signet of the Son of Man will stand forth in the eastern sky. The wise will then lift up their heads and know that the redemption of the Earth is near."*

If we *overestimate* the average human lifespan at 100 years, you can see that in the grand scheme of things, we are barely visible on the cosmic canvas. Yet in each human life lies the potential to reunite with *"Brahm,"*[11] to achieve the ultimate state of yoga, which gets us outside the circular room, expanding our individual limited consciousness into the Infinite Timeless consciousness of God. For, as Yogi Bhajan told us, "All things come from God, and all things shall return to God," including us!

Meanwhile while we're here on earth, we're bound by time. We ignore or forget that time is temporary. It is something man invented in order to measure distance, the space between things or events.[12] Of course, distance and time only exist within the created Universe, whereas the ultimate reality, and our true identity, is beyond Time and Space. Ideally, while we're here, we paint lovely scenes on the canvas of life, making it more beautiful, but we always want to be aware that they are, after all, just moving pictures!

Vedic scriptures described these four Yugas and gave the following mathematical computations. Together, the four Ages comprise one Maha Yug (Great Age) of 4,320,000 years. Two thousand Maha Yugas (8,640,000,000 years) are said to equal *merely* one day and one night in the life of Brahm (God).

# Yogi Bhajan: Man of God

MSS Shakti Parwha Kaur Khalsa

*"His teachings will save all mankind."*
*(Ashtapadi V)*

☬

Most people probably saw Yogi Bhajan as a dynamic, charismatic leader. They saw a giant of a man; they felt his powerful projection, piercing eyes, and a voice that penetrated deep into your soul. I saw all that, but I also saw his humility, the strength of his total surrender to God's will, and his acceptance and love for all people, even those who tried to discredit him. He was not your run-of-the-mill, mild-mannered textbook "sant." He was a true soldier-saint in the best tradition of his spiritual father, Guru Gobind Singh. He was a fearless advocate of Truth, and never failed to answer the call of duty, at the cost of his own personal comfort and even his health.

---

[10]  Dowling, Levi H. (1969) The Aquarian Gospel of Jesus the Christ. DeVorss Publications: Camrillo, CA, Chapter 157.

[11]  Wahe Guru, God

[12]  Movement requires space, there is distance between "things." Elementary particles (think about the atom) are always in motion. Everything in the created universe is in motion. Even apparently stationary or static things are "in motion," vibrating (just slower).

He encouraged and promoted everyone. He wanted others to excel and succeed. A Sikh in the highest sense of the word, he wished good to all, and competed with no one. I saw him sit patiently for hours while he was being verbally harassed and insulted. His response was simply, "God bless you." He never reacted. He was a man of action. "Don't react, resurrect" is one of his many quotable quotes.

Oh, he could roar like a lion when it was required, but let a small child, an innocent soul, enter the room, and he became gentle as a lamb. He always said and did what was best, not what was convenient or even popular. As a spiritual teacher he was a master. Being in his physical presence was always a powerful experience. Often all the mental chatter in our minds—fears, insecurities, neuroses, even questions we planned to ask him—would just evaporate, having been resolved on the spot or dissolved into insignificance. At other times, things we were holding below the surface of our awareness would be magnified so that our conscious minds would be forced to deal with them. While listening to him counseling someone, we would realize that his words were meant for us as well. Every word he spoke to us was a communication with our souls. Often the significance of a seemingly casual comment would become clear days, weeks or even years later.

He could lead us into incredibly deep, profound meditation, and afterward have us laughing and light-hearted. One of the greatest gifts of being in his presence was the way he always reminded us not to take ourselves too seriously—to lighten up, be light, and remember that all is part of God's play.

His basic premise was that God breathes in every body. He said it is everyone's birthright to be Healthy, Happy, and Holy, and he gave us the tools to claim it. For the first time in history, the technology of Kundalini Yoga was made public, and the consciousness of multitudes was awakened and transformed.

I am still amazed and awed by the miracle that was created during those thirty-five years he spent teaching in the West. Music, poetry, art, schools, *Gurdwaras,* and even businesses have emerged, and they all reflect the consciousness of Khalsa that he inspired and awakened within us.

From the very beginning, Yogi Bhajan made it clear that anything that he accomplished, any good he achieved was not his doing, but rather all credit belonged to his God and Guru. In the early days when he struggled and suffered, he saw the fame that was to come, and he wrote:

. . . . . . . . . . . . . . . . . . . . . . . . . . . . . . . . . . . . . . . . . . . . . . . . . . . . . . . . . . . . . . . . .

*"Some day the day shall come, when all the Glory shall be Thine.*

*People will say, 'It is yours.' I shall deny, "Not mine."'*

. . . . . . . . . . . . . . . . . . . . . . . . . . . . . . . . . . . . . . . . . . . . . . . . . . . . . . . . . . . . . . . . .

I was particularly fascinated with the way he referred to "my" God and "my" Guru, revealing an intimate and loving relationship based on personal experience. No one has been "converted" to Sikhism. We have simply found where we belong. We shall be eternally grateful to the Siri Singh Sahib for showing us the way, opening the door, and making us welcome. God bless him.

Sukhmani Sahib[13] tells us: *"It is only by great good fortune that one comes into contact with such men, from whom one learns the practice of the Name."* (Ashtapadi II)

And Ashtapadi VIII describes the Siri Singh Sahib perfectly:

---

[13] *Sukhmani Sahib:* "Peace Lagoon"; epic poem by Guru Arjan (used as the title of the book containing the Banis, daily Sikh prayers).

. . . . . . . . . . . . . . . . . . . . . . . . . . . . . . . . . . . . . . . . . . . . . . . . . . . . . . . . . . . . . . . . . . . . . . . . . . . . . . . . . . . . . . .

*"He makes no distinction between man and man:*

*His eyes rain nectar on whomever they fall…*

*He takes as his support the One alone, this God-awakened man:*

*He is imperishable.*

*With his mind he seeks humility.*

*His only pleasure is in doing what is good.*

*The man of God is not held by bonds,*

*But he keeps control over his wandering mind.*

*Whatever proceeds from him is good.*

*All those who are drawn into his company are saved.*

*Such a man of God is the support of the world."*

Chapter Two

# Dharma or Religion?

❁

## THE PURPOSE OF SIKH DHARMA

A dharma is a path or way of life. Sikh simply means "seeker of truth." Sikh Dharma is for those looking for the answer to the eternal question: "Who am I, and what am I here for?" Like all spiritual traditions, Sikh Dharma has its lineage and legacy, guidelines and philosophies, its heroes, masters and saints, and its history. It has a body of teachings and a technology. Sikh Dharma is a down-to-earth spiritual path for people to experience their own Divinity and Infinity.

Every human being is animated by a spark of the One Eternal Flame. We are the Light of the Divine contained in a human form. The human body is a vehicle given to us so we can travel through time and space on this planet to discover and experience that Divine Light in ourselves and in everything around us.

*"It's gracious to be humble. It's marvelous to be kind. It is loving to be compassionate. It's so human to be caring. There is no need for big philosophies."*

*—Yogi Bhajan*

Experiencing our own Infinite, indestructible, true identity while we are alive and functioning in our human bodies gives us unshakable fearlessness, love, and contentment. It enables us to face life honestly with courage and grace. A society of people who are conscious of the Divine Light within them and in everyone around them, and who recognize the inherent unity of all creation, form the foundation of a world of peace, prosperity, and integrity.

This is the vision and promise of Sikh Dharma. By service and meditation, we awaken to the everlasting Spirit of Love, the Divine Reality living within each of us, right now.

# *Why Sikh Dharma Is Not a Religion*

*By MSS Guruka Singh Khalsa*

*"Jesus came and left. Moses came and left. Guru Nanak came and left. Mohammed came and left. Everybody left, but nobody left. They all said the same thing, and they continue saying the same thing. They goaded people, they guided people, they climbed mountains, gave this sermon and that sermon, gave this counsel and that counsel. It is all cataloged and nothing has changed. Neither they have stopped trying nor have you stopped listening. It is a tug of war. Everybody has said the same thing from time immemorial to now. You have two ears, yet neither have you listened nor are you willing to listen.*

*"God told Guru Gobind Singh, 'Go and establish a path of righteousness. Let the human worship the Undying Being, the Akaal Purkh, not the dying being.' Jesus said not to worship idols yet I have never seen a single church where he is not hanging on the cross outside. Is that not an idol? Moses said to love all and worship one God, yet Jews feel they are the special chosen beings and everybody else is out. The Hindus were told to see God in everything. Their God is in their temple, sleeps at a certain time, and gets up at a certain time. Otherwise everything goes berserk. That is the hypocrisy of religion."*

*-The Siri Singh Sahib (Yogi Bhajan), 1977*

What is a Sikh? It is a very simple thing. "Sikh" means student. A student of what? A student of life. One who is here on this earth to learn how the universe works. The fact is, everyone is born to learn and understand reality. Everyone is born a seeker of Truth.

The word "religion" comes from the Latin "ligare," which means to tie or fasten. It has the same root as the word ligature or ligament. It means to be connected, tied. Doesn't that remind you of the word "yoga," which means to tie or yoke? To most of us, a religion is set of beliefs and practices. Just as **yoga** is not a set of postures but a **state of being in union with the One**, one can experience religion as being connected or tied to the One—to our origin and our Infinity.

Over the last 2,000 years, the concept of religion has degenerated from the real experience of union into a business where middlemen can collect money from people who want to know the truth of their own existence. Many organized religions are built upon the idea that you are separate from God and that you need someone else to intervene for you with that God who is "up there" so that you can be delivered from sin and redeemed.

Redemption, from the Latin "redimere," means to buy back again, to regain possession of what one has sold or lost. So what are we talking about? The soul has taken birth in this human form to attach itself back to the Infinity. Each of us is a part of God. The part of God in us is called the soul. So, we are here to merge with the totality. We are *already* One with God. We have simply forgotten. The experience of remembering is what we call redemption. It is regaining the knowledge, with which we were all born, that we are one with the One.

Dharma means the righteous path we follow in life. It is the way we conduct ourselves so that we can best fulfill our destiny. It is the spiritual technology we use; the foundation of our spiritual lifestyle, put into practice at every moment so that we can effectively fulfill our life's purpose.

Each of us has our own Dharma, although we may or may not realize it in this lifetime. Many people are spiritual 'window shoppers,' following first one Dharma and then another; however, as you awaken spiritually, your intuition guides you towards your own Dharma. The path that is perfect for you. When you experience it, you will know it.

All "religions" are of the past. In the future, there will be no such thing as organized religion. The concept of middlemen, such as priests and rabbis, will seem absurd. Each of us will stand as a sovereign spiritual, self-sensory human being consciously connected in the web of all existence.

· · · · · · · · · · · · · · · · · · · · · · · · · · · · · · · · · · · · · · · · · · · · · · · · · · · · · · · · · · · · · · · · ·

*"People will be open, straight, simple, and their beauty will be internal, not external. Men and women are going to reach out to each other with dignity, devotion, and an elevated loftiness of self. The beauty of the human character will be so bewitching, that not only will the ones who are willing become realized, but also their realization will be so profound that no destructive temptation by another person will be able to work. The Age of Aquarius will be the age of experience in which people of experience will be liked, respected, worshipped, talked to, and understood. It's not a matter of how old you are or how young you are or how white or how black you are. It is the fact that there is nothing more beautiful, more worthy, or more conscious than you."*

*-Yogi Bhajan*[14]

# Yogi Bhajan's Unique Contributions to Sikh Dharma

· · · · · · · · · · · · · · · · · · · · · · · · · · · · · · · · · · · · · · · · · · · · · · · · · · · · · · · · · · · · · · · · ·

### SS Gurukirn Kaur Khalsa

One of the most significant strands that Yogi Bhajan wove into his multicolored tapestry of teachings was that of the Sikh way of life. Being a Yogi, he dyed this strand with the special hue of living experience. The pattern that he created spoke to the souls in the West and fulfilled their longing to belong to the Guru. This was especially true with the unique contributions that he crafted in and around the Gurdwara service and environment.

---

[14]  © The Teachings of Yogi Bhajan, August 1, 2000; originally appeared in Self-Sensory Man

For those who had not grown up in a Sikh household and who perhaps did not even know what a Sikh was, explaining it in traditional religious terms might have been a bit of a "turn-off" to Western spiritual seekers. So Yogi Bhajan gave them practical explanations, as well as symbols and ceremonies.

One of the earliest symbols he gave was the Khalsa Flag, the traditional rectangular shape divided diagonally from upper left to lower right into two triangles, the lower one yellow and the upper one white. On top of these is superimposed a large blue *Adi Shakti* or *khanda*. This flag was first raised on a misty morning in 1972 at the Summer Solstice Celebration in Elk, California.

Yogi Bhajan described the significance of the flag, or *nishaan,* as follows: "Devotion is one-pointed emotions. You may try your best, but without *Bhakti* (devotion), there is no *Shakti* (power). Without *Shakti,* there is no *Bhakti.* That is why we make the Sikh Dharma flag half white and half yellow. The yellow represents *Shakti* while the white represents *Bhakti.* We fix a pole on this side and say the other side is the unseen pole of God. That is why one triangle comes from the heavens, and the other side comes from the pole side of the earth. We put the *Adi Shakti,* logo of infinity, on it. The triangle of the yellow is cut downwards; it represents the earth. The triangle of the white cuts upwards; it represents the ether. It is a union of earth and ether. That is our symbol. It is a symbol of *Raj Yog* (Royal Yoga). We are yogis, but we are kings of our domain. We are the princes of our own domain."[15]

This flag now adorns Sikh Dharma centers throughout the world.

From the very first days, Yogi Bhajan incorporated the stories of the Sikh Gurus into his yoga classes, and gradually shared practical facets of the Sikh way of life such as wearing a turban and maintaining uncut hair. He encouraged his students to incorporate and share these teachings in their own style, in a way that was meaningful to them. This trend is most apparent in the incorporation of the local language in various ways in the Gurdwara service, such as in the recitation of *Ardas* and translation of the *Hukam.* In many Sikh centers, the reading of the Guru in *Akhand Paths* is done with the translated version, including *Gurmukhi,* English, and Punjabi. The spread of Sikh Dharma throughout Latin America inspired a Spanish translation of *Siri Guru Granth Sahib.*[16] With the spread of the seed of Guru Nanak's message into different languages in countries worldwide, his teachings have truly blossomed into a universal faith.

---

[15] *Blue Skies of New Mexico,* 1975, page 149.
[16] Completed by Babaji Singh Khalsa of Mexico City in 2006.

It is through songs that Guru Nanak and those who followed him praised God's Name. Yogi Bhajan encouraged musicians to write songs about their personal experiences of spiritual understanding and about the courage and grace of Sikh heroes and saints.

Over the years, a remarkable body of work has been created. About the songs of the Sovereign Khalsa Spiritual Nation he said, "Sikh history cannot be understood any better than through our songs. It is lively, it is real, it is truthful. It shall continue to inspire millions. It is the language of the heart. It will be understood by people who understand the language of the heart. It will inspire humanity now and forever. It is descriptive, it is realistic, it is exact."[17] The children of the pioneers of Sikh Dharma grew up with such songs as "Guru Ram Das Lullaby" and "Ode to Guru Gobind Singh." Perhaps the best-known composition, "The Song of the Khalsa,"[18] was written by MSS Livtar Singh Khalsa of Atlanta, GA. In stirring terms, this song urges us to "Stand as the Khalsa, Strong as steel, Steady as stone. Give our lives to God and Guru, Mind and soul, Breath and bone." In many Gurdwaras, this song is always sung just before Anand Sahib.

Regarding the *Anand Sahib*, Yogi Bhajan adamantly opposed the conventional practice in most Gurdwaras of singing the fortieth stanza right after the first five. He explained that the structure of the composition created by the third Sikh Guru, Guru Amar Das, was a step-by-step progression toward enlightened consciousness. Singing the fifth stanza and then jumping to the fortieth would be like trying to jump over thirty-five stairs in a staircase. He considered it a great mistake to break the Guru's *bani* (sacred recitation) in such a way. Instead, he recommended either singing the first five stanzas and the *slok* or doing the prayer in its entirety.

During his lifetime, in his capacity as the Siri Singh Sahib, Yogi Bhajan usually gave a lecture in Gurdwara, wherever he happened to be at the time. These talks elucidated deeper points of meaning and clarified the practice of Sikh technology. Recordings of his lectures continue t on Sundays in a number of the major centers. In his words, "You need sociological, psychological, para-psychological understanding of the Guru.... Once you understand, you'll be up there."[19]

These talks emphasized the spiritual aspects and founding principles of Sikh Dharma, rather than the political, cultural, or social. Political speeches are avoided because they tend be divisive rather than unifying, secular rather than spiritual. He considered time spent in Gurdwara, in the presence of one's Guru, to be a very precious time for connecting to one's own soul and the Infinite. True to the origins of the faith, each soul is honored for its divine light. Such Gurdwaras avoid a sense of hierarchy based on position or status; gender, race, or age biases are not tolerated. Classes are given to train those interested in performing the Guru's *seva* so that anyone who feels the Guru's calling to serve is prepared to do so.

The Siri Singh Sahib regarded the Gurdwara environment as a special place for spiritual training. Key to this process is the practice of daily spiritual discipline, *sadhana*, which takes place in the early morning hours before the sun rises. In his teachings, Yogi Bhajan gave a sadhana, which begins with the morning prayer of the Sikhs, *Japji Sahib*, then a yoga kriya, over an hour of *Naam Simran*, mantra or meditation, and a short Gurdwara service. In this way, a person's day is set on a spiritual track from the beginning and that influence will color their actions and relationships throughout the day. Morning sadhana can be practiced in the Gurdwara sanctuary. Including the practice of yoga in one's daily spiritual discipline is considered to be

---

[17] © The Teachings of Yogi Bhajan, June 25, 1995; originally appeared in Khalsa Women's Training Camp Notes.
[18] See page 151.
[19] Personal Letter, March 17, 1997

honoring and caring for the body, which is the vessel for the soul, and one of God's greatest gifts. From early childhood, Yogi Bhajan was trained in the art of Kundalini Yoga and the practice of the Sikh way of life; within his body of teachings, these strands constantly intertwine. His unique weaving of these two traditions produced a fabric richly embroidered with the sacred threads of spirit.

# *Kundalini Yoga and the Siri Guru Granth Sahib*

········································································································

### *By MSS Shakti Parwha Kaur Khalsa*

Yogi Bhajan faced huge challenges when he began teaching Kundalini Yoga in the West. As a Sikh as well as a yoga master, he had to overcome ignorance on every front. Most of the students who came to learn had been taking drugs to get an experience of God, and he had to get them to try Kundalini Yoga instead, so they could have a spiritual experience without side effects, and without doing anything illegal. He had to instill the spiritual values he learned at the feet of his saintly grandfather in the undisciplined kids living the "go with the flow" and "let it all hang out" lifestyle that was prevalent in 1969 among the Baby Boomer generation.

Many Sikhs of Indian origin did not understand what Yogi Bhajan was teaching, and mistakenly assumed it was the sort of ritualistic thing that Guru Nanak had spoken against. Most people born into Indian Sikh families never learned the reasons behind the principles and practices taught by the Gurus. As a yoga master, Yogi Bhajan recognized the yogic technology found in the *Siri Guru Granth Sahib*, and the yogic wisdom with which the human Gurus were empowered. He opened up a whole world of meaning and practical application of the Guru's Words.

He explained the benefits of reciting the *banis*[20] – *not just as rituals, but as sound currents to enable us to receive specific experiences and the blessings with which they were imbued by their enlightened composers.*

In 1969, Yogi Bhajan created the Healthy, Happy, Holy Organization.[21] 3HO and Sikh Dharma have a symbiotic relationship. Although Sikh Dharma is legally a religion, more importantly, it is a way of life. 3HO Foundation is a separate 501(c)(3) nonprofit organization founded by Yogi Bhajan as a vehicle to spread the teachings of Kundalini Yoga and the technology of conscious living. 3HO Foundation is also a Non-Governmental Organization (NGO) in consultative status with the Economic and Social Council (ECOSOC) of the United Nations. People of many religions (or no religion at all) practice the teachings of 3HO. Not all Sikhs (especially Punjabis) practice Kundalini Yoga, and most people who follow the 3HO teachings are not Sikhs, though many of the first generation of teachers trained by Yogi Bhajan are. Again, these two technologies complement and supplement each other.

---

[20] Sikh's daily prayers: See Banis, page 86
[21] Incorporated in July 1969.

FOR THE RECORD:

## 3HO and Sikh Dharma

The Siri Singh Sahib knew that people who wanted to live according to the guidelines established by the Sikh Gurus would need a legal structure recognized by the United States government to protect their rights; for instance, to keep their hair, and wear turbans. So he facilitated the creation of the "Sikh Dharma Brotherhood" (later renamed "Sikh Dharma International") as a "religious Corporation," in other words a "church" organization. That way he could ensure that people who followed the path of the Gurus would be accorded the same rights and privileges as members of any other religion, both legally and administratively.

Chapter Three

# The Roots of Sikh Dharma

✦

## A BRIEF HISTORY

Over 500 years ago, Guru Nanak taught that Truth is a universal constant, and nobody has an exclusive right to it. Like the story of the six blind men describing an elephant, most of us have our own version of truth. Fortunately, there have been enlightened teachers like Guru Nanak who periodically come to remind us of the ultimate truth underlying the unity of humankind. They serve to awaken each of us to our own highest consciousness. Within the context of their historical time and space, these great souls have all taught the same universal truths of infinite consciousness. Many of these teachings became the foundation for the world's religions.

The Sikh path began in India when a man called Nanak said that people shouldn't fight about how to worship God. He proclaimed that there is One God, one universal Creative Energy, which pervades the entire creation (*ek ong kaar*), so we should **respect all religions.**

Guru Nanak saw God everywhere, in everyone. To him, everyone was equal in the eyes of God. At a time of widespread religious intolerance in India, Guru Nanak said, "There is no Hindu, there is no Muslim." This was a unique perspective, when Hindus were objects of scorn, suffering unspeakable persecution by the Mughal conquerors.

Those who followed Nanak's teachings, his students, were called *shishyas* or as we now say, "Sikhs." He was called Guru, a general term which means "Teacher." Actually, for Sikhs, the title of "Guru" is very specific, for only Guru Nanak and his successors are ever accorded that special title.

In the Hindu tradition, many spiritual teachers are called gurus. In the Western world since the 1960s, it was common to call any teacher from India who sets up shop on these shores a "guru." Now the term "guru" is used to describe your tennis instructor ("tennis guru"), or even your financial advisor ("money guru"). To Sikhs, the term is sacred, and can never be applied to anyone except Guru Nanak and his successors. Yogi Bhajan, a very devout Sikh, was very emphatic that we must never call him "guru."

## What is a Guru?

In Sanskrit, "gu" means darkness and "ru" means light. A "Guru" takes a person from the darkness of ignorance to the light of knowledge. So, the Guru is the one who enlightens you.

"Guru" in the Sikh tradition is an enlightened messenger of the Timeless. The Sikh Gurus served as reminders of the eternal wisdom, which is free from bigotry, rejects superstitions, dogmas and empty rituals, and emphasizes the value of a sacred life.

Guru Nanak was a Teacher whose words transformed and elevated the listener. He taught through the example of his life, and the words that flowed through him came out in exquisite poetry with mantric power. He formed analogies and comparisons to current happenings to educate and inspire people to discard superstition and empty rituals[22]. His words awakened rich and poor, peasants and emperors, Hindus and Muslims. Both women and men came to be his disciples, students of Truth, his *shishyas*. Thus Sikhs were born.

Over the period from 1469 to 1708, Guru Nanak laid the foundation for Sikh Dharma, and each of his nine successors added and expanded upon his teachings. By setting exceptional examples, the Gurus taught how to live spiritually fulfilling lives with dignity and honor while remaining active in the world.

The Tenth Guru, Guru Gobind Singh, formally enthroned the *Siri Guru Granth Sahib*, as the everlasting living Guru. It is the earthly physical container for the vibratory power of the Shabd Guru.

There is a saying, "Where you bow, there you shall be blessed." When a person bows to the *Siri Guru Granth Sahib*, he or she is bowing to the infinite sound current which holds the universe together, that which is beyond all personality, time, and space. It is the Shabd Guru, a compilation of words spoken by enlightened beings, and contemporaneously recorded for posterity.

The place where one feels humble before the Infinite is called the *Isht*. – It is the sacred spot where one bows one's head in reverence. It can be anywhere. It is personal. Some people climb a mountain, some go

---

22   Let us distinguish here between rituals performed by rote or habit, i.e., unconsciously, and ceremonial or sacred actions which are done with total attention and awareness.

deep into the forest, some go to church or temple or have an altar, or "sacred space" at home. The act of bowing gives the physical experience of surrendering, of "giving one's head," or mental chatter and personal ego to the Infinite Self. When we bow with humility and reverence to the Shabd Guru, it can create a space of deep openness and connection to the Infinite.

# What Do Sikhs Worship?

*MSS Guruka Singh Khalsa*

So what's up with bowing to a book and wearing turbans and all that stuff? It looks like a religion, but actually it is a technology--the spiritual technology of the future.

### Living Guru

Probably the most defining characteristic that bonds Sikhs all over the world is that we all worship the *Siri Guru Granth Sahib*, and only the *Siri Guru Granth Sahib* as our Guru. It is the compass that always points true North. It exists within everyone's heart. The Guru is that inner wisdom which takes us from darkness to light. We experience and accept the embodiment of the Shabd Guru, the *Siri Guru Granth Sahib*, as our only Living Guru. We don't bow to any living person as Guru.

The centerpiece of the community is the Gurdwara, where our living Guru holds court. So being in the Gurdwara is like being in the court of a King. There is a protocol. But at the same time, devotion is intimate, and in the Western Hemisphere, in any English-speaking Gurdwara (or Spanish, or Italian) anyone can read the *Hukam*, anyone can do the *Ardas* (prayer), and anyone can play *Gurbani Kirtan*. It only requires an attitude of reverence. (Before entering the Gurdwara, shoes are removed, and the head is covered. We wash our hands and bow before approaching the Guru.) There is a direct relationship between the Guru and the Sikh. Any Sikh can go straight to the Guru for guidance, without any intercessor. In Sikh Dharma there is never a "middle-man."

The beauty of our Shabd Guru is that it is impartial, impersonal, and always offers unbiased uncompromising guidance and inspiration.

The gist of the Guru's message, the essence of the teachings of Guru Nanak and his successors as embodied in the Siri Guru Granth Sahib is simply, "Chant God's Name. Live honestly with the conscious intention to make the world a better place for your having lived and breathed here, yet realize that everything here on Earth is temporary. Consciously connect with your own soul and with God by chanting His Name, by vibrating in the frequency of the Infinite, so it becomes your habitual state of consciousness, and prepares you to go Home[23] fearlessly and with joy. When the individual consciousness merges with the Universal consciousness, that divine union is a state of yoga. That is the goal of all yogas, and it is the purpose of life.

---

[23]   Home:  Everything comes from God, everything shall return to God (the Infinite Divine Light).

# A Convenient Truth: Ang Sang Wahe Guru

MSS Shakti Parwha Kaur Khalsa
and MSS Guruka Singh Khalsa

The Siri Singh Sahib once said, "The thing I like best about Sikh Dharma is *ANG SANG WAHE GURU*." I like it, too! It means that God is alive in every part of me. Every limb, every molecule, every atom is a manifestation of God. You might say it is a paradox. Despite my apparent human flaws or failings, this mantra acts as a reminder that God is living and breathing within me all the time!

This is different from the concept that "we are all born in sin; that we are separate from God." This idea of separation isn't my experience or my inner understanding. On one hand everything is God, and on the other hand we are impure, and God is pure? Yet unfortunately in many translations of the *Siri Guru Granth Sahib*, the word "sin" or "sinners" is used. Actually, this is not only a mistranslation, but also a basic misunderstanding.

"Sinner" is a concept that comes from the idea that we as humans are "unworthy." It is neither an accurate nor a useful descriptive term in the Aquarian frequency that we are now entering. As humanity evolves into its next level of consciousness the old concepts of guilt and sin are no longer relevant because they imply separation from the Infinite and create negative judgments of ourselves and others.

"*Paap*" as used by the Guru means any action that makes us feel alone and separated from God. "*Paap*" is not "bad." Nothing is good or bad, except that thinking makes it so. "*Paap*" is simply any action that pulls us into identifying with our ego and makes us forget our <u>true</u> identity, who we *really* are—Infinite, Radiant, Holy beings, and One with the Infinite.

The Mantra "*Ang Sang Wahe Guru*" is both an affirmation of identity and a joyous experience of one's own Infinite self. On February 11, 1990, the Siri Singh Sahib spoke about this as follows:

*"It is a fact of life that we are born in the image of God. Or else we conclude we are born in sin, and we have to work. There are two options: One option is that 5,000 years ago, man went through impulsations and convulsions—that's how he was born. Whether the egg came first or the chicken came first, nobody knows, but the fact is that there are two ways that reality is approachable…. One is (that) we are born in sin, we are terribly negative, we are condemned to death, we come here, we have to work hard, and we should give our money to the management and go home. That's one approach. Then the management will buy us a two-meter-square place in the heavens because they are better than us. So there is a middleman. We call it a priest or pundit. A middleman… A man who tells the commoner, 'You are good for nothing. You listen to me, and I'll elevate you. I'll get you to God. I guarantee it at the rate of $250 an hour. I'm a good man; I'm holier than you. You give me respect, you get under my control, and you listen to me. You are stupid, but if you listen to me you'll be better off.' It is called the evolutionary system of projecting my ego so that I am holier than you, and you are being a controlled audience, or it is called 'capture status,' and it has been going on for centuries…*

*"So basically what we have done is that something which is our moment-to-moment reality, which is our experience, which is our strength, we have made it commercial. We have made politics out of it. We have made a jurisdiction out of it. A science of infinity, a science of reality which is what religion truly is, that has become an individual telescope, bioscope, and situation through which man wants to show himself, or see himself on the planet earth. It has nothing to do with the state of consciousness we call heaven.*

*"But, there is a critical situation. And that is that the mind wanders. The wandering mind is not being controlled. You don't believe it? In the last 20 years there's not a great spiritual man on this earth whom I have not met or known, or understood. Even their minds wander. So, how to take a wandering mind, and make out of him a wonderful mind?*

*"This is the second option. This is all that the purpose of life is. This is all that life is about. To do it, you must talk to your own mind. And there is one mantra in Sikh Dharma that we use: 'Ang Sang Wahe Guru.'*

*"'Ang' means the limb; the part. We have a lot of limbs. We have ten trillion cells, and each cell has three parts "And 'Sang' is not your wife, your children, your friends, your houses, or your bank account balances. Sang is your mind. You know, if your mind goes berserk, everybody says 'goodbye' to you. There's not one person left. They take you to a mental hospital, and they put a straitjacket on you. I mean, you are the same person who was wonderful, appreciated, and loved, and everybody adored you, but you are rejected because your mind is off the beat. So 'Sang' means the mind.*

**Ed. note:** *nucleus, cytoplasm, and membrane) so, if you really want to know, we actually have 30 trillion limbs. That's how many 'you's' are within you.*

*"So, therefore, in this world of anxiety, it is a very straightforward situation. Whenever you feel depressed, or you feel angry, you feel empty, you feel shallow, or you feel abandoned; when you feel anything negative... you can only feel at that time that you are not true to the fact; Ang Sang Wahe Guru, God is alive within you!*

*"Because when we have the essence of this one single line: Ang Sang Wahe Guru, when we understand and experience it within all the realms of our tattwas — in our chakras, in our gunas, in our being, in our projections, in our rejections, in our pain, in our pleasure, and in our richness... when, in all that, we ALWAYS reach for Guru Ram Das[24], then there's nothing we should ever worry about. Our affairs will all be adjusted."*

# What Kind of Truth?

### By MSS Shakti Parwha Kaur Khalsa

Truth is an interesting concept. There are actually three kinds of truth. There's personal truth: what I personally believe as distinct from what you personally believe to be true—maybe they are the same, maybe not. But everybody has his or her own view of the world. Take any event seen by a group of people, and see how many different versions are reported. At the scene of an accident, each person believes his or her

---

[24]    The fourth Sikh Guru.  See page 100 for details.

version is the truth, yet they are seldom exactly the same. "It's all in the eyes of the beholder" certainly describes personal truth.

Personal truth is subject to change. Many of us change our belief system, our concepts and attitudes as we mature, get more information, and have more experiences in life—and that's okay. Personal truth can change.

Then there's relative truth: principles that people in general accept as true under certain conditions of time and space. We could say, "This is true under these conditions, but not under those conditions." Currently we accept the law of gravity as true. Though we may defy it by sending astronauts into outer space, still we don't deny it. We accept as fact that the Earth revolves around the sun. However, as you know, that belief wasn't always popular. There was a time when it was definitely believed that the sun revolved around the Earth. Let's not forget, the Earth used to be considered flat!

So personal truth and relative truth can change. However, there's the kind of Truth with a capital "T" that simply is. It's not subject to personal interpretation, belief, culture or bias of any kind. It is universal, ultimate, fundamental, unchangeable, and undeniably True. This is the kind of Truth that philosophers have been arguing about for centuries, that man has been trying to define, and preachers of many religions have been claiming as their own. It belongs to no one and to everyone. This is the Truth that is experienced in the deepest states of meditation and is, perhaps, impossible to completely describe with words. It is intrinsic within all things, but often eludes our view.

But that ultimate, infinite, unchanging reality, the actual Source of everything, isn't the personal property of anyone or any group, it is Universal. It has always existed, and shall continue to exist beyond time and space. That's the Truth that Guru Nanak taught when he said,

*Aad Sach*

*Jugaad Sach*

*Haibhee Sach*

*Naanak Hosee Bhee Sach*

☬

"True in the beginning,
True through all Time,
True even now,
Nanak says Truth shall ever exist."

Sat Nam means "Truth is your identity!" Thou art That! In other words, you are already an immortal divine being, temporarily here on Earth in human form to remember your divine identity, while learning to be human.

Chapter Four

# The Shabd Guru and the Sound Current

✴

## SINGING THE SONG OF THE SOUL

## Shabd Guru: Sacred Sound Current

*By MSS Guruka Singh Khalsa*

The Guru of the Sikhs is the *Siri Guru Granth Sahib*. The *Siri Guru Granth Sahib* is not a book. It is a container of the *Shabd*. The sound current of the songs in the *Siri Guru Granth Sahib* are known as the Shabd Guru. The Shabd Guru is not just a collection of uplifting, inspiring words written by enlightened saints, but a vessel of the sound current—the living Guru. By listening and experiencing this sound current, we understand that those who wrote these words transcended individual identity and ego.

Their words came from their unlimited exalted state of consciousness. Whenever we read, sing, chant or listen to these songs, we connect with our own excellence and our own infinity. There is no need to deal with any external human personality in this process. People have good days and bad days. They may be up or they may be down. But with the Shabd Guru, there is only a direct relationship with the Infinite. The Shabd Guru is a powerful technology, which is universally available to uplift and transform anyone in any walk of life.

Let's look at a deeper definition of Shabd Guru from its root structure. "Shabd" comes from Sha- and -bd. "Sha" means the ego, the attachments we identify with. "Bd" means to cut out/off, or to eradicate. The root meaning of Sha-bd is "that which cuts the ego." It is not just any sound. It is not even a wise sound or a song of truth. It is a sound that cuts away the ego that hides the truth from you.

In the Aquarian Age, ego will no longer work for anyone. The shift of the Age is changing the conditions of the mind. The Piscean consciousness operated with less sensitivity. You could hide actions, thoughts, and feelings with a high degree of short-term success. Some ego positions were favored above others in a family, society or environment. That has fundamentally changed in this new Age: all finite positions of ego are equally vulnerable.

We need to develop a new habit of awareness. We must learn an inner technology on which to base the identity of our Self in the Infinite. The Shabd Guru is the quantum technology that establishes that awareness. It is a compass point that directs us to the Infinite in each finite action.

The second word in the phrase Shabd Guru is "Guru." If we break this word to its inner *naad* or atoms of sound, it becomes Gu–Ru. "Gu" means darkness or ignorance. "Ru" is light and knowledge. "Gur" is a formula or instruction. A Guru then gives a Gur—a formula or technique—that transforms darkness into light, ignorance into knowledge, and the gross into the refined. A Guru then is an active knowledge. It is not the intellectual knowledge that simply classifies or analyzes. Guru changes you. Guru develops the capacity to see. It removes darkness and confusion.

The Shabd Guru transforms us by removing the barriers erected by the needs of the ego. The encounter with the Guru is through action. It gives you "Know How" not just "Know What." It gives you procedural knowledge that is in your cells and subconscious, not just representational knowledge in your ideas. To encounter the Shabd Guru is to learn by doing, by experience. The key practice of the Shabd Guru is the meditation and repetition of specific primal sounds and phrases.

Where do the patterns of the Shabd Guru come from? They exist from the beginning of creation. They are the tides and rhythms of the movement of the creative pulse of Infinite consciousness. They vibrate in all things continually. The ability to hear and feel them comes to a mind that is fearless, neutral, open, and awakened. The ten living Gurus and the many saints and *bhaktis* of the universal Sikh path heard them perfectly. They put that rhythm and pattern of energy into the poetic compositions of the *Siri Guru Granth Sahib*. That's why it is called a Granth rather than a collection. Granth means "knot." It is a knot that binds the pattern of awareness into the words of the songs.

Each Shabd is a template for an aspect of awareness and a potential of consciousness. Each Shabd is a kind of spiritual DNA that restructures the mind and stimulates the brain.

# How Do Sounds Affect Our Consciousness?

## The Science of Sound

### By MSS Guruka Singh Khalsa

There are 84 meridian points (similar to bundles of nerve endings) on the upper palate of the human mouth. One can feel that upper palate with the tongue and experience its different surfaces. Two rows of meridian points are on the upper palate and on the gum behind the upper teeth.

When we recite a mantra, our tongues touch these various pressure points in a sequence that stimulates the hypothalamus gland, which in turn makes the pineal gland radiate. People talk about the pineal gland secreting, but secreting hormones is only part of the story. The pineal gland is also sensitive to light. The great Chinese sage, Lao Tzu, called it "the gateway to heaven and earth."

When the pineal gland radiates, it creates an impulse in the pituitary gland, the master gland of the body (the gland that is the gateway to intuition). Think of a garage opener, for instance, where you press a series of numbers and then the * (star) key, and the door opens! Well, *mantra* is a key that opens the doors of inner awareness.

When the pituitary gland gives impulses, the entire glandular system secretes and a human being experiences bliss. This is the science.

"…The whole language of Gurbani has the power to make a person divine simply by reciting it correctly. One need not be concerned with its meaning in order to experience a change in consciousness. Bani has to be understood by the heart, not by the head. There is no power in the head. It is in the heart. The head is for God, and the heart is for you. That is why on that historic Baisakhi day[25] in 1699, Guru Gobind Singh asked for the head, and not for the heart. Whosoever lives with head to God and heart for self, that prayer is complete. The entire Siri Guru Granth Sahib is the calling of the lover for the Beloved. It is in naad."

*(Yogi Bhajan)*

---

[25] Baisakhi is the spring celebration of rebirth; see page 169 for more information.

# The Science of Naad and Gurbani

*Naad* means "the essence of all sounds." All languages contain sounds, which relate to one or more of the five elements of air, fire, water, earth, and ether. *Gurbani* is a perfect combination and permutation of sounds relating to all five elements in complete balance.

When Guru Arjan Dev, the Fifth Guru Nanak, compiled the *Siri Guru Granth Sahib* in 1604, he only put in those selections which were composed in *naad*. These compositions were called *Gurbani*.

# Syllable by Syllable:
# The Naad of Siri Guru Granth Sahib

*by Yogi Bhajan*

When we break up the words "Siri Guru Granth Sahib" into their *naad*, the syllables of each word tell the essence of the meaning of *Siri Guru Granth Sahib*. Every word has a *naad*, and every *naad* has a combination.

Siri means the entire light of the sun's creativity, Lakshmi[26]. Whatever has been created, whatever shall possibly be created or can be created, is called *siri*, "great."

Guru ("Gu" means darkness, and "ru" means light) means from darkness to light, from ignorance to knowledge. Guru is one who gives you the technology to remove your ignorance.

Granth ("gra" means knot, "an" means ultimate, and "naath" means owner, master, God) is that which creates the ultimate knot with God. Anything which creates the ultimate knot with God is called a granth. Granth is not a book and can never be a book. Sahib ("saa" means "light," infinity, and "hib" means "now") is the totality of here and now.

# Experiencing and Understanding Gurbani

*by Yogi Bhajan*

The Guru's Word *(Gurbani)* is what the Guru spoke. It is the imprint of the essence of God. It is the pathway to Infinity. If the ordinary human being speaks it, it will always elevate him to that state of consciousness of the Guru. The Guru's consciousness is united with God, so the person will automatically get united with God if he speaks the same words. It is a scientific and direct way to unite the finite with the Infinite Consciousness. The hypothalamus will get the same tingling. The impulses of the pituitary will function the same way and get the other glands to secrete also in the same way as it was in the body of Guru Nanak.

Gurbani is nothing but a total, illustrated, facilitated science of naad for human knowledge. It is an individual effort. Read Gurbani in the way Guru says it, understand it, and you will be in such ecstasy, you will not believe it! Concentration on the construction of the word and the sound is the proper way to recite Gurbani. As you are creating the sound, the meaning will automatically come to you, now or later. It is just a matter of time and space. You must listen to your own construction of the Gurbani. This is the technical way in Naad Yoga.

---

[26] Goddess of Love and prosperity.

There are two ways to go about understanding *Gurbani*. The first is to know the meaning through purposeful study; and the second is to recite it, and you will automatically understand the meaning intuitively. *Gurbani* has to be recited with the tongue, through *japa*. But, when you read meditatively for the purpose of understanding the meaning, it is okay.

# The Power of the Shabd, Gurbani Kirtan and Nam Simran

## Mind Control

When we can control our mind we can create great things, because the power of the mind is also very unlimited. When disciplined and focused, it can change the vibrations and the magnetic psyche of the earth. That is why we do *kirtan* (singing of God's praises). *Kirtan* literally charges the magnetic psyche of the universe with those vibrations of the Word of the Guru, the *naad*, and creates a state of ecstasy.

## Nam Simran

*Nam simran* is continuous remembrance of one's True Identity through repetition of the names of God. *Nam Simran* is required to prepare for *Gurbani* to have its effect. It is the complete science of the Word and sound. It changes a human's biological and psychological metabolism of his or her body, mind, and soul.

# Conscious Sounds

Conscious speech has the power of invocation. We can literally create reality through the power of our words. Every word we speak is an act of creation, yet we may not understand our own power.

Breath is God's gift of life, and when we use it to utter sounds, those sounds carry the creative power of the universe within them, setting up a chain reaction in the cosmos. Everybody knows the saying, "Be careful what you pray for, you're liable to get it!" That's good advice. It's also a very good idea to be conscious of what we say all the time, because the words we choose plant vibratory seeds that sooner or later must sprout—for better or for worse.

Having a mantra going on in your head, or out loud, allowing your breath and all the rhythms of your life to "chant God's Name" is extremely practical advice.

# Sat Nam: What Does It Mean?

Here's a marvelous mantra you can use. It is more beneficial than "Aloha"—and can be used in practically every circumstance. It's just two syllables. SAT NAM. rhymes with "but Mom"—(unless you're Canadian or British.)

*Sat Nam.* I always begin any correspondence or conversation with these two syllables, which mean: "Truth is God's Name" and/or "Truth is Our Identity." By saying this, I establish, however briefly, instant rapport, a common ground respectfully acknowledging our shared divine identity—certainly an excellent basis for any intelligent conversation! Following that initial greeting, we are free to disagree about other things such as the best restaurants, movies worth seeing, the latest fashions, or even politics and religion.

I say *SAT NAM* to my accountant, my banker, and my non-Sikh relatives. I've programmed my answering machine greeting so that it begins with *SAT NAM*. I'll never forget how Yogi Bhajan made fun of our usual American greeting of "hello." He pronounced it, "Hell – oh." — I got the message.

## Sat Nam and Wahe Guru

*"Sat Nam is the shabd in which you have superiority over God. God is a slave in the hand of the devotees. Sat Nam purifies the entire time and space whenever you speak it, even if only once; it does not matter when. It is the "superior self-power of God."*

*(Yogi Bhajan)*

*Sat Nam* is the *bij mantra* or seed sound, which can elevate the consciousness of any person to Infinity, and *Wahe Guru*, is a mantra of ecstasy, which can bring the experience of that Infinity.

Loosely translated *Wahe Guru* means, "Wow! God is Great! Indescribably terrific!"

*Wah* means Infinite, *he* (pronounced *hay*) means Thou, and *Guru* means Self (the Divine Teacher within). When *Wahe Guru* is chanted, it brings you very near God.

## Sa Ta Na Ma

*Sat Ta Na Ma* is called a *panch shabd* (*panch* means five, since it actually contains five primal sounds). When you separate SAT NAM's syllables into the *naad, s(aa)* means Infinity; *t(aa)* means birth; *n(aa)* means death; and *m(aa)* means rebirth or resurrection. The "aa" sound puts the projective energy into each component and is considered the fifth sound.

# Frequently Chanted Mantras and Shabds

*"Mantram siddhyam, siddhyam parameshwaram"*

He who masters mantra, masters God Himself.

Chanting is not singing it is not talking; it is *vibrating*. All mantras should be chanted from the navel point, unless otherwise instructed.

## Mul Mantra (Mool Mantra)

The opening lines of *Japji Sahib* by Guru Nanak, "Mul" means "root"

| | |
|---|---|
| EK ONG KAR | One, Creator, Creation |
| SAT NAM | True Identity |
| KARTA PURKH | Doer of Everything |
| NIRBHAO | Fearless |
| NIRVAIR | Without Revenge or Anger |
| AKAL MOORAT | Image of Deathlessness |
| AJOONEE | Unborn |
| SAIBANG | Self-illumined |
| GUR PRASAAD | Guru's gift |
| JAP | Repeat |
| AAD SACH | In the beginning: Truth |
| JUGAAD SACH | Through the ages: Truth |
| HAIBHEE SACH | Even now: Truth |
| NANAK HOSEE BHEE SACH | Nanak (says) Truth shall exist forever. |

- Hiss the "ch" sound of each *"sach"* with emphasis.

- *There must be a space* (not a breath, just a space) between the words AJOONEE and SAIBANG. Do not run them together. (Emphasis on the EE sound will help to avoid running the words together.)

. . . . . . . . . . . . . . . . . . . . . . . . . . . . . . . . . . . . . . . . . . . . . . . . . . . . . . . . . . . . . . . . . . . . .

*I am one with the One Creator and this is the gift of that One True Guru.*

*The Creator of all is One,*

*Truth is His Name,*

*He is the Doer of everything,*

*Fearless and*

*Revengeless,*

*Undying, (the image of deathlessness)*

*Unborn and*

*Self-illumined.*

*This is revealed through the True Guru's Grace.*

. . . . . . . . . . . . . . . . . . . . . . . . . . . . . . . . . . . . . . . . . . . . . . . . . . . . . . . . . . . . . . . . . . . . .

## Subtle Differences - Impact Result

"Jappa means repeat….There are two sounds which you must remember. One is…'Aad Such, Jugaad Such, Haibhee Such, Naanak, Hosee Bhee Such.' That is part of the 'Mool Mantra.' That is whenever you are shaken, it will fix your root, spontaneously….And, suppose you are stuck, can't move: 'Aad Such, Jugaad Such, Haibhay Such, Naanak Hosee Bhay Such.' Anything which is stopping you shall give the path. Mantra moves the elements. Mantra moves all five elements, plus heavens, plus Earth."

"Try to chant so that it will have impact. Do you know what I am saying? … What is *Gurbani*? It is a permutation and combination of sound current."

*Yogi Bhajan*

## Kundalini Shakti Mantra:
## Ek Ong Kar Sat Nam Siri Wahe Guru

*Ashtang Mantra  (Eight-part)*

| | | | |
|---|---|---|---|
| *EK*: | One | *NAM*: | Name |
| *ONG*: | Creator | *SIRI*: | Great |
| *KAR*: | Creation | *WAHE*: | Beyond description: "Wow!" |
| *SAT*: | Truth | *GURU*: | Dispeller of darkness or "Teacher" |

# The Technology of of Chanting "Long Ek Ong Kar"

*Two-and-a-half Breath Cycle:*

Sit with a straight spine and APPLY NECK LOCK (raise chest, pull chin straight back).

1. Inhale deeply and chant Ek Ong Kar (One Creator [created this] Creation)

Ek is short and vibrated powerfully at the Navel Point (not shouted).

Ong is long and chanted in the back of the throat. It vibrates the upper palate, and comes out through the nose.

Then slide into Kar for the remainder of the breath.

2. Inhale deeply again and chant Sat powerfully from the navel point followed by Naam (Truth is His Name) until you're almost out of breath, then

REACH for the S'ree (Great), which is a short syllable at the end of the breath.

3. Inhale only ½ breath and chant Wah-hay G'roo (Wow! Great Dispeller of darkness and ignorance).

Wah is short. Hay is extremely short and briefly precedes the Guru, which is pronounced G'roo, almost as one syllable and using up the rest of that ½ breath.

Inhale deeply again to repeat the cycle. Continue for at least 7 minutes.

This mantra was the first, and almost the only mantra Yogi Bhajan taught during his first year in the United States. It is extremely powerful and energizing when done correctly. It opens the chakras. These syllables are the "code" letters, or you might say they are the phone number of the direct line to "connect" you, the creature, with your Creator.

The ideal, most effective time of day to chant this mantra is during what are called "The Ambrosial Hours," the 2 ½ hours before sunrise in the morning.

Long Ek Ong Kar's are done for 7 minutes as part of the Aquarian Sadhana.

It has been said that a person can attain liberation by chanting this ashtang mantra correctly, for 2 ½ hours before sunrise for 40 days. ("Correctly" means with full concentration, accurate rhythm and proper pronunciation.) Try it, you will be amazed!

Other suggested time periods for personal practice of this mantra are: 31 minutes or 1 hour. Chanting it for 2 ½ hours can give you a marvelous experience.

# Dhan Dhan Ram Das Gur

This is the shabd (sacred sound current) to chant when you need a miracle. It is in praise of Guru Ram Das, the fourth Sikh Guru, the "Lord of Miracles."

*Dhan Dhan Ram Das Gur*

*Jin siriaa tineh savaari-aa*

*Pooree hoee karaamaat aap sirjanhaaray dhaari-aa*

*Sikhee atay sangatee parabrahm kar namaskaari-aa*

*Atal athaaho atol too*

*Tayraa ant na paaravaari-aa*

*Jinee too(n) sayvi-aa bhaa-o kar*

*Say todh paar ootaari-aa*

*Labh lobh kaam krodh moho*

*Maar(i) kadhay todh saparvaari-aa*

*Dhan so tayraa thaan hai*

*Sach tayraa paiskaari-aa*

*Naanak too Lehnaa too hai*

*Guru Amar too veechaari-aa*

*Gur dithaa taa(n) man saadhaari-aa*

☬

Great, Great is Guru Ram Das.

Whosoever has heard him, has become perfect.

The miracles have perfected themselves:

God Himself has come in and prevailed through this manifestation.

Your Sikhs, and the entire Sangat (congregation) bow,

And revere You as the Supreme Lord.

You are Unshakable, Unfathomable, and Immeasurable.

Your Extent is beyond limit.

Those who serve You with love

Are carried across the world-ocean by You.

Greed, attachment, lust, anger and ego —

You have beaten and driven out these five passions.

Honored is Your Place,

True are Your Bounties.

You are Nanak, You are Angad

And You are Guru Amar Das —

So do I recognize You.

Seeing the Guru, my soul is sustained.

(Page 968 in *Siri Guru Granth Sahib*, "uttered by Rai Balwand and Satta the drummer.")

## Ardaas Bhaee Amar Daas Guroo

. . . . . . . . . . . . . . . . . . . . . . . . . . . . . . . . . . . . . . . . . . . . . . . . . . . . . . . . . . . . . . . .

*When you want to insure that your prayer will be effective, preface it with this mantra. It is also helpful to chant to keep the ego from taking control of a person when a certain stage of yogic progress has been attained.*

. . . . . . . . . . . . . . . . . . . . . . . . . . . . . . . . . . . . . . . . . . . . . . . . . . . . . . . . . . . . . . . .

*Amardaas Guroo Ardaas Bhaee*

"Guru Amar Das confirms the prayer has already been answered."

*Raam Daas Guroo, Raam Daas Guroo, Raam Daas Guroo*

"Guru Ram Das, the Lord of Miracles, covers the prayer in the past, present and future."

*Saachee Saahee* means "True Ink." Yogi Bhajan translated this as Guru Ram Das's "Seal of Truth," guaranteeing the prayer.

## Ek Ong Kar Sat Gur Prasad, Sat Gur Prasad, Ek Ong Kar

If you want to change negativity into positivity, this is the mantra to use. It is recommended to chant it five times in succession. It is infinite and removes all thoughts of the little self.

> *"I translate it this way 'I know that I am One with God. This is the True Guru's gift. The knowing comes by grace. It is a gift from the Guru within you.'"*

> (MSS Guruka Singh)

## Gur Mantra: Wahe Guru

Wahe Guru Wahe Guru Wahe Guru Wahe Jio

# My Introduction to the Siri Guru Granth Sahib

### MSS Shakti Parwha Kaur Khalsa

One of the first things Yogi Bhajan did, soon after we met at the East West Cultural Center,[27] was to lead me to its library. He reached way up high to the top bookshelf, and carefully lifted down a large volume he called the *Siri Guru Granth Sahib*. Reverently opening to the first page, he asked me to start reading. I began with the words of Guru Nanak. "There is One Creator who created this creation, Truth is His Name. He is great beyond description…" I read a few more lines, and then I said, "I'm really not interested."

He gently closed the volume and replaced it on the shelf. It was at least six months later before I read from the Guru again. Only by that time I had learned a little more about this remarkable "Shabd Guru" and had gained some understanding of the power and wisdom it contains. Yogi Bhajan had explained that all the words in it were spoken by men who were in a state of divine union with God, their individual consciousness merged with the universal consciousness (a state of "yoga"), and what they said in this state of bliss was written down and preserved intact. Their words of divinely inspired poetry were captured in a 1,430-page volume called the *Siri Guru Granth Sahib*. He emphasized that this volume is not a history, not a "bible," not a "book," but words of revealed truth, to be shared and experienced by anyone who reads or hears them. We can say, in fact, that Sikhs worship the Word of God. Containing writings of six Sikh Gurus, as well as saints and seers from all walks of life, from tanners to bean sellers, Hindu, Sufi, and Muslim alike, the *Siri Guru Granth Sahib*, the Shabd Guru, is the living Guru of all Sikhs, now and forever.

## About the Siri Guru Granth Sahib

The *Siri Guru Granth Sahib* was compiled by Guru Arjan, the fifth Sikh Guru, in the early 1600s. This amazing *Shabd* Guru was the first interfaith and universal scripture (see Ed. Note below). It is a collection of religious, mystic, and metaphysical poetry written or recited between the 12th and 17th centuries in the Middle and Far East, and it is made up of poems or songs composed in *naad* using the *ragas* of classical Indian music. The compositions come from a diverse group of holy men, saints, sages, and bards from many different cultural traditions (Muslim, Sufi, Hindu, and Sikh), from various social positions, and are written in several different languages including Sanskrit, Prakrit, Rajasthani, Persian, Arabic, Bengali, and Marathi. These were all recorded in the Gurumukhi script. Because of this, this diverse collection of divinely inspired poetry is accessible to anyone who learns the Gurumukhi script and can be accurately recited in the correct *naad* of the original composition.

---

[27] Then located at Ninth and Vermont in Los Angeles, California.

**Ed. Note:**

*It is difficult to describe the Siri Guru Granth Sahib without calling it a scripture, yet "scripture" is a misleading term, inferring it is only relating stories of past history. The term "scripture" does not describe the mantric power of the words on its 1,430 pages. However, to explain to someone who has not experienced the sound current of the Siri Guru Granth Sahib, who sees merely a volume of printed pages, and is told these pages are considered more than sacred, I suppose calling it a "scripture" may help to open the discussion.*

The *Siri Guru Granth Sahib* holds a profoundly uplifting, expansive, powerful frequency expressed through the sound current of its *naad* and enhanced by the meanings of the words and the universal message of its poetry. When approached with reverence and devotion, and especially in a collective or group meditative state, it can uplift us, heal us, and guide us into the future.

Yogi Bhajan taught that when we chant in a group the power and vibratory effect for each participant is multiplied exponentially. For instance, when ten people chant together, each gets the benefit of one hundred people chanting!

It is important to remember that everything in the *Siri Guru Granth Sahib* was contemporaneously recorded. These are not versions of events told many years later, in stories told by people who were not there at the time. They are accurate verbatim transcripts of what was spoken and sung by its various authors. One of the Sikh Gurus disowned his son because the son agreed to change one word in the *Siri Guru Granth Sahib* to appease and please the Emperor!

# My Experience Reading from the Guru

## By MSS Shakti Parwha Kaur Khalsa

Yogi Bhajan went back to visit India in 1972. He had become spectacularly successful in America and Europe as a Kundalini Yoga teacher as well as a highly respected Sikh leader. Sad to say, success can bring jealousy and resentment, even in the realms of so-called "spirituality." There had been attempts on his life, and plots to detain him in India and prevent his return to the U.S. He wrote me: "I may not come back alive. Please pray for me."

So, what to do? When his letter reached me, I remembered how much he had emphasized the power of the Shabd Guru, what tremendous faith he had in "his" Guru, so I thought, "Well, he believes in this *Siri Guru Granth Sahib*, so we should set up a continuous reading." I rallied the 3HO community, and we signed up, taking turns reading in tandem, one or two hours at a time, 24/7, to keep up a continuous sound current. We didn't know anything about the protocol for *Akhand Paths*. We didn't know that we should change the *ramalas* at the completion of each complete recitation. We just kept on reading, and when we got to the end, we started all over again without a break. We continued this for ten days until Yogi Bhajan's safe return to California.

I had signed up to read every day from 4 p.m. until 6 p.m. None of us in Los Angeles had yet learned to read *Gurmukhi*, so we all read in English. It was not easy. Sitting that long wasn't comfortable, and sometimes the formal British–English (not American-English) translation seemed awkward, but the amazing thing was the effect that the reading had on me. At that time, my job involved dealing with the public—and I hated it. I was frustrated and annoyed most of the time. The strange thing was that as the days passed, I noticed I was getting mellower and mellower, calmer and calmer at work. Things that used to bother me just didn't seem to matter. I wasn't reacting to what people said and did. I simply wasn't getting upset. That was my first experiential confirmation of the power of the Guru, and the effect on one's life the recitation of its sacred words can have.

# A New Perspective

The Guru's words gave me the gift of a new perspective on life. I began seeing and recognizing the relative unimportance of most day-to-day annoyances in the context of the "big picture." There's a line in the "Song of the Khalsa"[28] that speaks about seeing the world "through the Guru's eyes…"

The Guru tells us over and over that this life is temporary, and the only thing we can do that is of permanent value is to chant God's Name. Chanting and remembering God's Name gives us a way to experience God's presence here and now, so that when the time comes to leave this physical body and take the journey Home to Him, we will be comfortable—in familiar territory.

It is interesting to me that it's not just Sikh Gurus whose words are quoted with this main message (preserved verbatim, by the way, transcribed into the *Gurmukhi* script), but also Hindu, Sufi, and Muslim saints and poets—all of whom were enlightened.

But there's more to it than that. Yes, intellectually as we read the inspired words of the *Siri Guru Granth Sahib*—even in translation—we see the world and its events in the greater context of Infinity. On a subtler level, and even more profoundly, by reciting these words, we put ourselves into the same vibratory frequency as the enlightened beings who originally spoke them while they were actually in conscious divine union with God. That union is a merger known as "yoga." Surprisingly, repeating their words elevates us even when we recite in English.

I must say, however, that when I finally learned to read in *Gurmukhi*, it became an even more dynamic and transformational experience. That's because of the mantric power of these sacred syllables. An actual physiological transformation takes place when we recite mantras as they were originally spoken.

When we recite portions of this "mantra," we are re-recording on our subconscious minds, thus erasing undesirable pre-recorded programs. The higher vibrations of the Guru's Word intelligently and automatically dissolve the vibrations (thoughts and feelings) of fear, insecurity, anger, jealousy, hatred, and resentment that prevent us from experiencing the joy of our own divine soul. It may not happen overnight, but I guarantee you, if you consistently read aloud from the *Siri Guru Granth Sahib*, you will get a broader, wiser, and actually more practical view of life, relationships, the world, and your place in it.

You don't have to be a "Sikh" to read from the *Siri Guru Granth Sahib*. Anyone can approach the Guru, and if you approach humbly with reverence and a willingness to open yourself to the experience and guidance of the Guru, you will most certainly be uplifted. As Guru Nanak was a Guru for the Aquarian Age, similarly,

[28]  *Song of the Khalsa*, page 151

the Shabd Guru is a timeless guide, available to all people, with no strings attached. You don't have to join anything, or commit to anything (except during an *Akhand Path*, when you have to commit to keep reading until the next reader takes your place, since it is a continuous reading).

Our Shabd Guru is always available, never has a bad mood or a toothache, and has no personal favorites among us. The Guru's wisdom and guidance is impartial, universal, and asks nothing in return.

When I met Yogi Bhajan I wasn't expecting to join any group. I just wanted to be happy. I wasn't even looking for God, and certainly wasn't planning to become a member of any religion, but reading from the *Siri Guru Granth Sahib* gave me an experience I could not deny. This was something real, something that made my life smoother, happier, and more meaningful.

I'm basically a skeptic. It is the experiential aspect of Sikh Dharma that makes me live it and love it. My faith in God and Guru has developed and continues to grow stronger because of the experiences I have day after day. Yogi Bhajan said it best, "Doing is believing." All I know is, it works for me.

# Things to Know About Reading from the Guru

## Protocol

As in many traditions, we take off our shoes and cover our heads before entering the Gurdwara. Out of respect, before approaching the *Siri Guru Granth Sahib* to read, we wash our hands. It is customary to bow, and make an offering. As you prepare to read during an *Akhand Path*, the current reader continues to read aloud, and you simultaneously read along with her/him for a line or two as you slip into place, so that the continuous sound current of the recitation is not interrupted.

## Identifying the "Authorship"

It was the custom of those times for a poet to include his own name in his works. As you read, you'll find many sections that include the phrases, "thus speaks Nanak" or "Nanak says." At first you think, "Wow, Guru Nanak wrote this whole thing!" But actually, he didn't, though he contributed many verses. Something written by the Fifth Guru doesn't say, "...thus spoke Guru Arjan Dev," but rather, "Thus spoke Nanak." Because all the Gurus realized it was the same divine light of inspiration, the same consciousness of Nanak that flowed through each of them. So every section written by one of the six Gurus included in the *Siri Guru Granth Sahib* acknowledges Nanak as its author. Sections by Kabir and other *Bagats* are signed with their own names. You can tell which Guru actually authored a section by the number used, such as *Mehela Pehla* (First Guru) or *Mehela Panjavan* (Fifth Guru), indicating it was from the First (Guru Nanak) or Fifth (Guru Arjan), etc. Strangely enough, Guru Gobind Singh didn't include any of his own writings in the *Siri Guru Granth Sahib*. His words can be found in several of the daily prayers Sikhs recite, and in a volume called the *Dasam Granth*.

# FACTS ABOUT THE SIRI GURU GRANTH SAHIB [29]

- The Guru Granth Sahib contains hymns of thirty-six composers written in twenty-two languages, employing a phonetically perfected *Gurmukhi* script.

- The Fifth Guru, Guru Arjan Dev, who compiled the first version, composed 2,216 of the 5,894 hymns.

- Besides the hymns of other Gurus, he also included 937 hymns composed by fifteen saints and eleven poet laureates of the Guru's court. Hindus, Muslims, Brahmins, and "untouchables" all come together in one congregation to create a truly universal scripture[30].

- The *Siri Guru Granth Sahib* was composed in poetry, perhaps to prevent alterations and/or adulterations, and to appeal to the human heart. Further, poetry can always be interpreted to suit changing cultures.

- It includes material originally written or spoken in Sanskrit, Prakrit, Rajasthani, Persian, Arabic, Bengali, and Marathi. The phonetically complete *Gurmukhi* font meets the need for inscribing a multi-linguistic scripture that is also musical.

- Music forms the basis of the rhythms and classification of the hymns, using Indian *ragas*. This form is used not only to preserve the originality of the composition, but also to provide a divine experience through the medium of music and the primal sounds of God's creation. The Gurus themselves created some of the thirty-one *ragas* used. Several hymns use popular folklore and meters.

- The Holy Granth verses are often sung as *kirtan* to reveal true meaning directly through cosmic vibrations. The melodies bond the listener to the spiritual light of universal intelligence.

- This was the first interfaith and universal scripture. It is a compendium of religious, mystic, and metaphysical poetry written or recited between the 12th and 17th centuries in Mid-Eastern and Far-Eastern continents.

---

[29] Excerpts from "Spiritual Uplift With Gurbani" article by Professor Harbans Lal, from the *Times of India*, Saturday, October 19, 2002.

# Getting the Guru's Personal Advice:
# Taking a Hukam

### By MSS Shakti Parwha Kaur Khalsa

As a mother I felt terribly guilty for the way my son James' life had turned out. Although Yogi Bhajan had assured me many times that it was not my fault, still I felt responsible.

After a fifteen-year separation from James, I was shocked when I saw him again. He had gained a huge amount of weight, and even worse, when I visited his apartment, I was horrified when I saw the conditions in which he was living. Paper bags overflowing with old newspapers were strewn all over every room, and there were other signs of abnormal housekeeping.

He had met his wife, Lucille, at an outpatient rehab center shortly after he had been discharged from the Army. Although he had gotten well, she hadn't. His wife was a mental patient. He was her legal conservator. James told me that frequently in the middle of the night she would try to commit suicide, and he would have to call 911 and get her to the hospital for treatment. When I visited their apartment, it was one of those times, so she wasn't there.

When I got home, I was terribly upset. In tears, I phoned my dear friend, Dr. Sat-Kaur Khalsa. She is not only the Secretary of Religion for Sikh Dharma International, she is also a professional Marriage and Family counselor. I told her what I had just seen and how disturbed I was about James.

She listened to my story and then suggested something I could do if I wanted to get guidance and clarity about my son and his situation. She said, "Write down the whole story: your relationship with James, and how you feel about it. Then when it is all down on paper, go to the Gurdwara, say an *Ardas*, and then take a *Hukam*.

On my next day off (I remember it was a Thursday), I sat down at my typewriter (this was many years before I had a computer) and started writing. I typed and cried, and cried and typed some more. I kept on typing with tears streaming down my face until I had written pretty much the whole scenario: my marriage at 18, James' birth at 20, my divorce at 22, James taking drugs when he was 18 (and having a bad trip on LSD) while I was in India, his enlisting in the Army where, after two days, he attempted suicide and went AWOL, then my receiving his letter saying he was planning to go to Canada.

It was at that point in time, December of 1968, that I met Yogi Bhajan who said to me, "Your son's in trouble isn't he?" When I said, "Yes," he said, "I can help you." And so he did. He told me "There's nothing more powerful than the prayer of a mother for her son, and if you will chant this mantra (*EK ONG KAR SAT SIRI WAHE GURU*) for one hour every day for 40 days, before sunrise, your son will be all right."

It worked. Actually, it only took about ten days before I heard from James, and he came safely, if not sanely, back to Los Angeles.

Then after a few days, James left town, and I didn't hear from him again for fifteen years. When I next saw him, and met the woman he had married, and then saw how they lived—well, I needed a way to deal with my feelings. So I did what Sat-Kaur suggested.

As soon as I got it all down on paper, I went to the Gurdwara, made an offering, said a prayer, and then I took a *Hukam*.

The Guru absolutely spoke to the situation. The words confirmed what Yogi Bhajan had told me years ago! The *hukam* said that even in the mother's womb, it is God who is responsible for the life of every soul. I wish I had written down the exact words, but the message was quite clear. It was sufficient to ease my guilt (it certainly verified what Yogi Bhajan had told me), and demonstrated that the Guru's words can supply whatever answers we need, whenever we need them. I went home and burned the document I had typed. No need to go over the past again.

# How to Take a Hukam

Anyone can take a *Hukam*. A *Hukam* is the "order of the day." It is the Guru telling us what to remember and understand in order to guide our lives and put our circumstances into perspective. The procedure is that after covering your head and washing your hands, you stand and offer a prayer, make an offering, and bow your forehead to the ground, then go and sit behind the *Siri Guru Granth Sahib*. After chanting a few lines of an appropriate *shabd* or mantra, meditatively asking for guidance, you reverently open the pages of the *Siri Guru Granth Sahib* at random. When you see the first section or shabd that begins on that page, read it. It is the Guru's direct message to you.

A hukam is understood with the heart, not the head. Let the Guru's words penetrate and the meaning will become clear; you don't have to 'figure it out.'

The *Hukam* should be read out loud and clear with the understanding that you are conveying the Guru's powerful pronouncement. It is the Guru speaking directly to the *Sadh Sangat* giving an order, an instruction to be meditated upon and taken to heart. So the reader sharing the Guru's words needs to speak with firmness and conviction.

 At Guru Ram Das Ashram in Los Angeles, we write down the first and last lines of each *Hukam* taken at every Gurdwara, so that anyone can locate the full passage later.

# How I Learned to Read Gurmukhi

### By MSS Shakti Parwha Kaur Khalsa

Having experienced the wonderful effect that reading in English from the *Siri Guru Granth Sahib* had on my disposition and peace of mind, I thought it might be a good idea to be able to recite the words in *Gurmukhi*, the original language in which the Shabd Guru was written. This was easier said than done, because for some reason I had a huge mental block. However, by the grace of God and Guru, and thanks to the infinite patience and kindness of Bhai Sahib Dayal Singh[31], who taught me *Gurmukhi* and didn't give up on me, I eventually learned.

I was really, really slow! After sadhana every morning he would sit patiently as I stumbled painfully through *Japji Sahib*, syllable by syllable. In the beginning it took me two hours to read the whole thing. Without his encouragement and patience, I might have given up.

Now I can easily read it in less than five minutes. Actually, the *Gurmukhi* alphabet is quite simple, totally phonetic, made up of only 42 letters, so really, anyone can learn to read it. Certainly if I could do it, anyone can!

The *Gurmukhi* script makes it possible for everyone to read all the selections in the *Siri Guru Granth Sahib*, even if they were originally written in Persian or Sanskrit, Arabic, Bengali or some other language or dialect.

I don't think I could have learned from anyone other than Bhai Sahib. He was indeed a saint. Despite my tedious, slow pace, he never let me feel stupid. He kept encouraging me every step of the way, God bless his soul! Anyone who knew him will never forget him.

Once I had gained a relative proficiency, I used the *Akhand Paths* as a training ground for reading in *Gurmukhi*. During the hour I had signed up for, I would read in English as fast as possible for about 30 or 40 minutes (and I'm a really fast reader) and then practice reading in *Gurmukhi* for the rest of the time. Little by little, my pronunciation improved. I felt that the Guru was actually teaching me, and continues to do so. Reading in *Gurmukhi* I experienced what is called the *rasa*, the "taste" of the Guru's words. It is delicious! As I've explained, when we recite the very words that came from men who were in a state of divine union with God, our tongues are accessing the exact same meridian points on the upper palate as theirs, and so we are attuned to the same vibratory frequency; our consciousness is blessed and uplifted.

Anyone can learn to read *Gurmukhi*. (If I could do it, anyone can!) If you are interested, find a Gurdwara, or a minister of Sikh Dharma and ask for help. Or, on the Internet, go to

http://sikhism.about.com/od/learntoreadgurmukhi/Learn_Gurmukhi_and_Sikh_Prayers_Online.htm

You can start by learning the alphabet, clearly described on this site.

---

[31] Bhai Sahib Dayal Singh: see "My Experiences with Death" to learn more about him.

## THE MOOL MANTRA IN GURMUKHI

| | |
|---|---|
| ੴ | *ik ong kaar* |
| ਸਤਿ ਨਾਮੁ | *sat naam* |
| ਕਰਤਾ ਪੁਰਖੁ | *kartaa purakh* |
| ਨਿਰਭਉ | *nirbha-o* |
| ਨਰਵੈਰੁ | *nirvair* |
| ਅਕਾਲ ਮੂਰਤਿ | *akaal moorat* |
| ਅਜੂਨੀ | *ajoonee* |
| ਸੈਭੰ | *saibhang* |
| ਗੁਰ ਪ੍ਰਸਾਦਿ | *gur parsaad* |
| ਜਪੁ | *jap* |
| ਆਦਿ ਸਚੁ | *aad sach* |
| ਜੁਗਾਦਿ ਸਚੁ | *jugaad sach* |
| ਹੈ ਭੀ ਸਚੁ | *hai bhee sach* |
| ਨਾਨਕ ਹੋਸੀ ਭੀ ਸਚੁ | *Nanak hose bhee sach* |

# Yogis in the Siri Guru Granth Sahib

### By MSS Guruka Singh Khalsa

*Ed. Note:* *The poem called "The Yogi," by Guruka Singh Khalsa, was originally published in "Furmaan Khalsa, Poems to Live By" by Yogi Bhajan.*

Many yogis lived in India at the time of Guru Nanak. They lived alone, they did not marry, nor did they work for their living. They lived in meditation caves, wore large earrings (to indicate that they heard only the Word of God) and coats made from rags patched together (to indicate poverty), and carried a begging bowl, a cow horn, a purse, a deerskin (to sit on for meditation), and a walking staff. With their unwashed and uncombed, matted hair and their bodies covered with gray funereal ashes (to remind themselves of the constant presence of death), they practiced their yogic disciplines and lived apart from the villagers and common householders. They begged for their food, and ate only what they were given.

Guru Nanak's meeting with such yogis is recorded in the *Siri Guru Granth Sahib* in a section called the "Siddha Gosht." Many hymns in the *Siri Guru Granth Sahib* address the yogis and make it clear that those who lived the lifestyle described above were not true *yogis* at all (that is, those who are united with God and live in that state of Union), but simply caught up in rituals and self-righteousness.

The poem below was written at the request of Yogi Bhajan, right after I completed the translation of the *Furmaan Khalsa,* in which Yogi Bhajan signs himself as "the Yogi" in most of the poems.

He asked me to read the entire *Siri Guru Granth Sahib* and extract *every* reference to a yogi, yogis or yoga, and then create an "epic" poem describing all of these qualities. I found exactly 108 references to yoga and yogis!

This then is the epic poem "The Yogi" as requested by Yogi Bhajan. It incorporates all of the 108 qualities of a Yogi as described in the *Siri Guru Granth Sahib* and describes Yogi Bhajan's identity as "The Yogi" in the Guru's words.

# "THE YOGI"

The Yogi fights the only battle worth fighting
He kills the five demons[32] and sends them to hell.
By winning this battle he saves his whole family,
And he saves everyone in the world as well.

Night and day he lives awake,
He lives in a trance of pure delight.
In love with the One, he lives without fear,
And prays to serve only the One great Light.

He has the most priceless gift of all…
He's satisfied—he lives at peace.
Deeply content in God's meditation,
He sits detached, in sweet release.

He is the master of his mind.
While others feel themselves apart,
While others are wishing and hoping,
He contemplates God within his heart.

He lives in the house of unspeakable bliss
And is ever happy with the gift of God's love.
He treats all people just the same.
No one below, no one above.

How can the Yogi do this?

Everything he sees is God,
He sees the Truth in everything.
In everyone, in every place,
In every sound he hears it ring.

---

[32] Lust, Anger, Greed, Pride, Attachment

He enters through the open door,
He makes the home of God his own,
He hears the music of the spheres,
His mind is pleased, his Way is known.

He wears the pure white robe of Nam.
He lives a life that's filled with Truth.
He lives in wedded bliss with God.
He lives a life of self-control.
He lives aware of all that flows
In and out of all nine holes.

He walks the path of righteousness.
His mind is shining like the sun.
He feels at home in all three worlds,
And is a friend to everyone.

He travels deep within himself.
He cleans himself from inside out.
And bowing at his inner shrine,
He worships God within his mind.

His mind is steady, clear, and true,
No need to fight, no need to argue.
What he says and what he means are one and the same.
He's the master of his mind. He remembers the Name.

He is modest and kind, truthful and sweet.
He shares his virtues with all whom he meets.
He understands God's Inner Command,
And sees the actions of God's own hand.

*With his mind immersed deep in the One,*
*Free from doubt… natural, pure,*
*He takes his seat in God's true home,*
*And makes the will of God his own.*

*With a gentle touch, he controls his thoughts.*
*He is ever alert in body and mind.*
*He forgets himself, yet lives alone.*
*He knows this world is not his home.*
*He calls no single thing his own.*
*Moving easily through all the spaces*
*He gains True knowledge, sees many faces.*
*He lets go of his wanting, anger, and conceit.*
*He needs little sleep and little to eat.*

*He eats just simple, natural fare.*
*Lives in balance, at ease, content.*
*His heart lotus is open wide.*
*He understands the Guru's Word,*
*And merges with the God inside.*

*He is filled with God.*
*He holds fast to the root,*
*Sips nectar from the breast of life,*
*And lives in peace, beyond all strife.*

*Living deep…*
*Close to the core,*
*Breathing…*
*Breathing …*
*Nothing more.*

*The Yogi knows the way of the heart.*
*Wearing earrings of silence, he hears it all.*
*He follows the royal path of Raj Yog.*
*He ever serves the True Guru,*
*And easily sees what's false and True.*

*The whole world is his wallet*
*Filled with kindness for all.*
*His walking staff is the One God's Name.*
*His bowl is full of God's meditation,*
*And he sees all places and beings the same.*

*He sits on the deerskin of the five elements*
*And the whole world comes to his door.*
*He roams freely through the city of his body,*
*His vision awakened, his heart at home.*
*While storms are raging all around,*
*The winds of desire just leave him alone.*

*He lives at peace through all the four ages,*
*A brother and friend to all saints and sages.*
*He is master of the earth, air, water, and fire,*
*He roams through the ethers, lower and higher.*

*The Yogi is master of the cosmic sound*
*Wherever he sits there is music around.*
*He finds his horn in the star flung realms.*
*The unstruck sound is ever new.*
*He sings the glories of God and Guru.*

*Music always fills his mind.*
*For the yogi's horn is God Himself,*
*God is the sound ... God plays the tune.*
*His heart-sun enters the house of the moon.*

He plays upon the untouched strings,

Vibrating… music of the spheres,

All tones merging into one,

The voice of God is what he hears.

His mind and breath are the gourds of his veena,[33]

His fingerboard is the One True Lord,

On the strings of his heart, He plays clear and sweet.

He lives forever free from joy and sorrow

And uses today to create tomorrow.


His mind is ever steady, though the winds of change blow strong.

His mind is ever clear, filled with music of the spheres.

He doesn't praise or slander anyone.

He knows that "good" and "bad" are just a game.

To him pure gold and common iron are both spirit, just the same.


God is his personality. God is his form.

He's beyond separation, death, and sorrow.

He keeps his lower self restrained.

In him, all virtues are contained.


He wears the earrings of the Word.

His coat is woven of forgiveness.

His bowl is full of universe and stars.

Awareness is his walking stick.

He knows that God is never far.


To live in the constant presence of God

Is the ashes on his body.

His job is to ever praise the One.

His religion is the Guru's Way.

He longs for God all night and day.

---

33   Veena: stringed musical instrument

He kindles the fire of Divine vision,
With the fuel of his body and the bellows of love

He burns all his doubt and smears the ashes on his body.
He lives in the warmth of that Divine flame
And ever begs for the One Lord's Name.

In Divine knowledge, concentration, and Sangat
He is ever awake, with love in his heart.
With the needle of meditation and the thread of God's Word
He lives to practice his most divine art.

He remembers the bright Lord and merges his soul.
Union with God is his only goal.
He slays the five demons, keeps God clasped to his heart,
Remains fixed in God's love, and is never apart.

He sees the One Lord in the moon and the sun.
He sees God's light within everyone.
He sees God in the forest. He sees God in his home.
Full of awe … full of wonder … he is never alone.

All his rituals are drowned in singing God's praises.
He dwells on the Name and begs for none else.
By Guru's grace he is blessed with the highest respect.
God removes all his doubts, and unites him with Him.
God lives in his every fiber and limb.

His trance is true freedom and release from the world.
Beyond sloth and desire, anger and pain,
His body and his senses serve him,
And his Way of life is the love of the Name.

*Indescribable joy is the food which he eats.*

*He ever leans on the staff of Truth.*

*His mood is one of contemplation.*

*He practices the yoga of God's meditation.*

*He stills his ego and sings the Lord's praise.*

*He reflects on the essence of All ... night and day.*

*He sits in the fearless, timeless place,*

*And loves to gaze on the playful Lord's face.*

January 21, 1988
Columbus, Ohio

# Chapter Five

# Daily Practice: Three Things to Do and Four Tools to Use

✪

## THE TECHNOLOGY OF SIKH DHARMA

T**he Sikh Way of Life is very simple.** It is based on three things to do, and four fundamental tools to help you do them.

# *Three Things to Do*

. . . . . . . . . . . . . . . . . . . . . . . . . . . . . . . . . . . . . . . . . . . . . . . . . . . . . . . . . . . . . . . . . . .

1.  **NAM JAPA** – Get up every day before the sun rises and meditate on God. "He who calls himself a Sikh must wake up early in the morning before sunrise and meditate on the Divine."

    – Guru Ram Das

    Yogi Bhajan used to say, "Any fool can sleep through the sunrise, but wise is he who wakes up before the sun." He explained that during those "ambrosial" hours (*first vela*), from 4 to 7 a.m., the solar energy is at the correct angle for us to "catch the wave" and ride that solar energy into the day. Get up late, and you've missed the wave.

    To prepare for meditation, Yogi Bhajan recommended taking a cold shower (*ishnaan*). This "hydrotherapy" strengthens the nervous system, stimulates blood circulation, and clears the *aura*.

    Yogi Bhajan also included in our morning spiritual practice (sadhana) the practice of Kundalini Yoga, the Yoga of Awareness, to balance the body, mind, and breath.

    Meditating on the One God, chanting God's Name to clean the mind—and singing with joy—to feel uplifted and divine.

2.  **DHARAM DI KIRAT KARNI** – Earn your living by working honestly by the "sweat of your brow" to support yourself and your family. Speak the truth and deal with everyone honestly, never begging or "wheeling and dealing," and simply serving and being grateful for the work that God gives you.

    Guru Nanak advised his Sikhs to marry and raise a family, to be householders and create cozy homes. A Sikh can be single or married—with children or without. He or she can be a student, or practicing a profession. In work life and in social life, we strive to remember with every breath to be aware of God in our hearts and in the whole creation.

3.  **VAND KE CHAKNA** – Live generously and share what you have rather than keeping it all for yourself. Be kind and wish well to everyone. Inspire and elevate others. Respect the right of each person to practice their faith on whatever path they choose.

    Protect the weak, and serve your community and humanity as a whole. Welcome everyone into your home, and feed and serve them with love.

    Whenever you enter the house of a Sikh, you can be sure to be offered food and drink within a few minutes. Sikhs love to feed people!

# Free Kitchens

The *Langar* or free kitchen was started by the first Sikh Guru, Guru Nanak Dev. The tradition of langar expresses the ethics of sharing, community, inclusiveness, and oneness of all humankind. It was designed to uphold the principle of equality among all people regardless of religion, caste, color, creed, age, gender, or social status. At the Guru's Langar anyone and everyone was welcomed and fed. Everyone sat together, no one higher or lower than anyone else, no matter to what caste they belonged. Kings and beggars sat side by side on the ground together. In fact, before being permitted audience with the highly revered Guru, even the mightiest potentate had to first sit and eat with everyone else.

Today, there are free kitchens provided by Sikhs all over the world, and every Gurdwara serves langar after the service. And, of course, everyone is welcome.

# Giving in the Name of God

Yogi Bhajan once said that the main job of a Teacher is to teach people to give. He encouraged his students who had dropped out, to go back to school, prepare for careers, get jobs or start businesses so they could thrive, prosper, and earn enough to be able to give generously. He pointed out that God is the greatest (and the only) Giver, and so the more we are able to give, the more godlike we become. He was generous even in the early days in America when he had practically nothing. Still he gave, at every opportunity.

# Buying One Pencil

One evening, early in 1969, when Yogi Bhajan had finished teaching a class at the East West Cultural Center in Los Angeles, he was walking with Dr. Judith Tyberg and a few of the students to get something to eat at the Ontra Cafeteria on Vermont Avenue when they came upon a blind man selling pencils. The Yogi proceeded to give the man all the money he had just earned—just for one pencil! Dr. Tyberg was horrified. At the Cafeteria, she asked him how he expected to pay for his dinner. He didn't say anything. When he had filled his tray and was standing in line for the cashier, a student—who had not even been in that evening's class—ran up to him and eagerly paid for his dinner!

# *Four Tools to Use*

## *Bana, Bani, Seva, and Simran*

BANA is the distinctive style of clothing worn by those committed to the Sikh path. Our *bana* is our outward projection. It includes uncut hair and beards, our turban, and for many of us, the wearing of modest white clothing. *Bana* is a reminder to act consciously, because when you stand out and look regal, your behavior must match up to your appearance.

BANI refers to how you speak. How do you communicate? What is your body language? What's your spoken language? Is it graceful? Is it inspiring and uplifting? Is it direct and loving? Bani is when the frequency of your communication is divine. Reciting the powerful syllables of the *banis* (daily prayers), and singing/chanting the sacred songs written by the Gurus, provides automatic self-cleaning of the subconscious mind and help us to constantly focus on the Infinite with every breath.

SEVA is selfless service: actions done to serve others without expectation of payment or reward. Seva is a state of being in service to humanity. You do service, not as the finite you, but as the God in you serving the God in others. That's the beauty of seva. We strive to constantly be awake for opportunities to be of service.

SIMRAN is constantly reminding oneself of one's own divine identity through the use of mantra and meditation. With the tool of *simran*, one can see the God in all. Meditating on the words of the Shabd Guru and chanting those Sacred Sounds (mantra) facilitates the experience of our own Divinity. Simran trains our minds and senses to recognize—and remember—the Divine Light within us and in all of creation, and to live based on that knowledge and experience. This creates inner peace.

To help us be in the state of *simran*, we avoid intoxicants in any form. We are vegetarians and do not eat meat, fish, poultry or eggs. Why? Because they are difficult to digest, produce toxic byproducts in the body tissues, and as a matter of awareness that "you are what you eat." We do not use drugs (except when medically necessary), alcohol or tobacco. It is common knowledge that smoking can cause lung cancer, and alcohol destroys the liver. We don't want to pollute the body, and we don't want to become addicted or attached to external substances that alter consciousness. The technology of Sikh Dharma can bring the experience of ecstasy without the risk of addiction or side effects.

## *Chanting God's Name*

"In the Beginning was the Word, and the Word was with God, and the Word was God." Sound familiar? Well, the foundation of Sikh worship is simple: nothing in this world is permanent, so remember God's Name, the sound current of the Infinite, and connect yourself with what is real. This will help you remember your divine identity here and now, and will naturally come to your lips when you die, so that your soul easily reunites with your Infinite identity, with God. Repeat, recite, chant, and remember God. This is the main message of the *Siri Guru Granth Sahib*.

# The Names of God

*SAT NAM, WAHE GURU, HAR, HAREE, HARAY, RAM*—there are many names of God, and many mantras containing various names of God. The Vedantists say, "God is One, men call him by many names."

God's Name vibrates within every breath you take. The Guru (*Siri Guru Granth Sahib*) guides us, reminds us, inspires us, and elevates us to rise to that awareness.

Let's explore these tools a bit more, starting with *bana*, the noticeably distinctive clothing we wear.

# Bana in a Western World

### By MSS Guruka Singh Khalsa

Yogiji was passing through Columbus, Ohio, and about a dozen of us went to the airport to be with him during a two-hour layover. As we sat in the terminal, Yogiji, dressed in his long white robe and turban, closed his eyes, and stretched out his long legs. We all knew better than to assume that he was sleeping.

Suddenly, an American businessman barged into our midst. He was immaculately dressed in a perfectly pressed three-piece suit and tie, carrying a briefcase, and wearing shiny, expensive shoes. Looking rather indignant, he approached Yogiji, and said in a loud annoyed voice, "What are you?!"

Yogiji slowly opened one eye and looked the businessman up and down. Then, closing his eye, he said, "A human being."

Annoyed, the man responded, "Yes, I know. But where are you from?"

Yogi replied without opening his eyes, "Venus."

Now the fellow was getting really annoyed. "But what kind of clothes are those?"

Yogiji opened both eyes... wide... and carefully scrutinized the man up and down before answering the man's question with another question, "What kind of clothes are those?"

"These are normal American clothes!" the man replied.

"No," said Yogiji, "Don't you know that those are British clothes?"

Indignantly, the man said, "Well, what kind of clothes are you wearing?"

Yogiji closed his eyes and settled himself comfortably. "These," he said with a slight smile on his lips, "are the clothes of the future."

# Bana: Looking Different

By MSS Shakti Parwha Kaur Khalsa and
MSS Guruka Singh Khalsa

As a thirteen-year-old boy, Gobind Rai saw most of a huge crowd of Sikhs run away in fear after witnessing the beheading of his father, Guru Tegh Bahadur, the great martyr to the cause of religious freedom. The boy was determined that when he became the Guru, his Sikhs would not be cowards. In 1699, as Guru Gobind Singh, he created the Khalsa (pure ones). To ensure their appearance would always make them recognizable as Sikhs, he gave them the gift of *bana*, a way of dressing that is an unmistakable display of Sikh identity and all that it stands for. Just as firemen, policemen, nurses, and clergy wear clothing that immediately reveals who they are and what service they provide to the public, similarly Sikhs were given a uniform! Of course, as with every part of Sikh Dharma, our "uniform" is also a spiritual technology, which strengthens our awareness of ourselves as divine beings.

The form of a Sikh is simple. Uncut hair covered with a cloth turban and a steel bracelet (called a *kara*) worn on the wrist. Many Sikhs also wear a *kurta* or *chola*—a loose-fitting tunic over *churidars*—pants that are loose-fitting around the thighs and buttocks and tight around the ankles, and a *cummerbund*—a cloth wrapped around the mid-torso region to maintain mild pressure on the solar plexus and internal organs.

We keep our physical form as the Creator created it, not removing or cutting hairs from any part of the body. A Sikh will not alter his or her body except for medical necessity.

# The Spiritual Technology of the Turban

By MSS Guruka Singh Khalsa

From the time of the first Sikh Master Guru Nanak, tying a turban was part of the unique spiritual path that would become Sikh Dharma. For thousands of years, in many different spiritual traditions, the turban has served a unique and universal purpose. It helps a person to experience, integrate, and maintain his or her highest consciousness throughout the day.

## How Does The Turban Work?

The top of the head, the place where babies have their "soft spot," is called the Tenth Gate. In yogic terms, it is also known as the crown *chakra* (the Seventh Projected Energy Center of Consciousness). Thousands of years ago, yogis and spiritual seekers discovered that the hair on the top of the head protects the Tenth

Gate from sun and exposure. In addition, the hair acts as antennae, absorbing and channeling the energy of the sun into the body and brain. To amplify the effect and direct the radiant energy into a spiritual focus, spiritual seekers would coil or knot their uncut hair at the top of the head at the Tenth Gate – also called the solar center of the head.

In men, the solar center is on top of the head at the front (anterior fontanel). Women have two solar centers: one is at the center of the crown *chakra*, the other is on top of the head towards the back (posterior fontanel). For men and women, coiling or knotting the hair at the solar centers focuses the energy upward to higher centers of consciousness and helps retain a spiritual vibration throughout the day.

This hair knot, traditionally called the "rishi" knot or *joora*, assists in the controlling and directing of energy in meditation. In ancient times, a "maharishi" was someone who could regulate the flow of energy in the body, meditatively and at will. The rishi knot assists in the channeling of energy in meditation (*Naam Simran*). If one cuts off the hair, there can be no rishi knot. By giving us the rishi knot and the turban, the Sikh Masters shared a very ancient technology for how an ordinary person can develop the capacity of a Rishi.[34]

The next step after tying a rishi knot is to put on a turban. There is a technology to wearing a turban. More than a religious symbol of commitment, it actually helps concentration, because when tied correctly, the pressure of the multiple wraps keeps all the bones of the skull in place and activates pressure points on the forehead that keep a person calm and relaxed. Turbans cover the temples, which is said to help protect a person from mental or psychic negativity. The pressure of the turban also changes the pattern of blood flow to the brain. And, of course, it protects the hair from dust and dirt. You feel clarity and readiness for whatever you may face during the day.

# *Turbans*

By MSS Guruka Singh Khalsa (posted on SikhNet)

Throughout history, the cutting of hair has been associated with the taking of power. Conquerors would cut the hair of the conquered as part of their enslavement. In Sikh Dharma, there are no slaves and no masters. Each person lives to his or her highest excellence, and treats others as equals. The *bana* (clothing) of a Sikh who has taken *Amrit* is the visible manifestation of the belief that each person is sovereign, noble, dignified, and divine, and that no human being is higher or lower than any other human being.

For many, hair is sexually attractive. By covering our hair we can keep from stimulating the sexual nature of those who are not our spouses. It is up to each of us to maintain our purity and integrity.

The Divine Energy that governs the Universe and guides our own life is mostly unknown to us. It is mastery as well as mystery. Living with an awareness of that Divine Energy within oneself and the entire creation allows us to live in our highest potential. Covering your head is an action of acceptance that there is something

[34] Kundalini Yoga The Flow of Eternal Power by Shakti Parwha Kaur Khalsa - Perigee Trade; Perigee edition (August 1, 1998)

greater than you and shows your willingness to stand under that greatness. Covering your head is also a sign of humility, of your surrender to God, and only to God. It is a technology of understanding—of standing under

Wrapping a turban every day is our spiritual practice and declaration that the highest, most visible part of us, this head, this mind, is dedicated to our Creator. The turban becomes a flag of our consciousness as well as our crown of spiritual royalty. Wearing a turban over uncut hair is a technology of consciousness that can give you the experience of God. This experience is for everyone, men and women alike.

# American Women – and Turbans

*By MSS Shakti Parwha Kaur Khalsa*

The Siri Singh Sahib often repeated that until women are respected, there would be no peace on Earth. He made it one of his priorities, part of his "mission" to remind women of their strength, their grace, and their responsibility to the human race. He established Khalsa Women's Training Camp where he lectured and taught extensively every summer for many years, empowering each woman by reminding her of her nobility and her cosmic role as a woman, as a divine *Shakti,* to nurture and inspire all of humanity. Such Women's Camps are still being held all around the world as women share his transformational teachings.

In 1972 Yogi Bhajan led a group of eighty-four yoga students to India where many of them decided to take *Amrit*; in other words, to formally commit to live as *Khalsa¹* Sikhs. [35]

I had stayed in Los Angeles to "hold the fort," and teach Yogiji's Kundalini Yoga classes at Pitzer College in Claremont, the North Valley YMCA, and at the Melrose and Robertson classroom. Here's the way I heard the story about what happened in India.

Yogi Bhajan guided the group to the bottom of the steps leading up to the *Akal Takhat* where the ceremony was to be performed, but he didn't lead them any farther. He didn't even go along with them. He left them there. They had to climb those steps and take their vows independently of him.

At the conclusion of the ceremony, all the men were presented with turbans. Whereupon the women in the group, Americans of course, protested that they should also be given turbans to wear. After all, they had heard that "Khalsa knows no gender." So all the newly baptized *Khalsa* returned to the United States "crowned" with turbans. The men had the new name of Singh (lion), and the women had the name *Kaur* (princess).

---

[35]   See "Becoming Khalsa" p. 169

# *My First Turban*

. . . . . . . . . . . . . . . . . . . . . . . . . . . . . . . . . . . . . . . . . . . . . . . . . . . . . . . . . . . . . . . . . . . . . . . . . . . . .

### *By MSS Shakti Parwha Kaur Khalsa*

I wasn't yet wearing a turban, but one afternoon, in the living room of Guru Ram Das Ashram on Preuss Road, Yogi Bhajan was saying that wearing a turban was really important to reinforce the growing collective identity of *Khalsa* and to show support for his work in bringing Sikh Dharma to the West.

So, I picked myself up, walked home (only a block away at the time), and wound several white *chunis* (delicate white silk scarves) around my head in the best version of a turban I could create, leaving a couple of inches of fabric hanging down in back like a short tail.

When people pointed out that there was something "left over" hanging down from the turban, I said, "I like it that way." Yogi Bhajan kind of laughed, saying that was the way the Nihung Singhs tie their turbans! (The Nihungs consider themselves to be the army of Guru Gobind Singh and are universally known for their fierce bravery in battle.)

Once I tied that first turban, I never stopped wearing one in public, though I eventually dispensed with the Nihung style. I got some cotton fabric to use as an under-turban, and then wound silk material around that. It's quite a meditation to wind those five yards of fabric into a head covering that won't come off. I found that it helped to add a *chuni*, several yards of sheer fabric that drapes over the turban, shoulders and chest, and then attach a decorative turban pin to keep the over-*chuni* from flying off. Yogi Bhajan told us that without the final over-*chuni*, it's just a "work" turban. Only royalty were allowed to wear the graceful over-*chuni*, which amplifies a woman's arcline and enhances her grace and subtlety.

# *Turban Styles*

Women's turban styles have evolved since the early 1970s, when they were piled so high they resembled stovepipes. Keeping them on was a challenge. I remember driving several of the staff members to a movie one afternoon in my classic 1960 Cadillac. (It had fins. We called it the "Big White Whale.") Every time we hit a bump in the road, my turban bounced up higher and higher uncovering my ears. So I had to hold it down with one hand and drive with the other.

Then there was the turban (not my style) that was worn pushed far back on the forehead, revealing hair parted in the middle and swooping down on either side toward the temples. For a while I wore a *chakra*—a

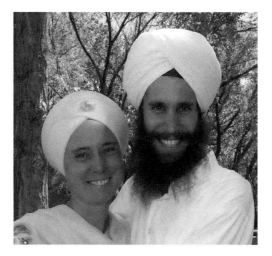

circle of steel near the top of the turban. Although some women are adept at using the cotton fabric to cover the top of the head, I never mastered that art, and instead after the turban is wound and the *kanga* (wooden comb) inserted, I tuck in a crocheted "doily."

The turban is the crown of spirituality, the symbol of the regal heritage and legacy of Guru Gobind Singh. One of the greatest insults to a Sikh is to knock off his turban. Yogi Bhajan showed the men how to tie a "battle turban" that is quite firmly secured.

## How to Tie a Turban?

SikhNet has a collection of videos on how to tie different styles of turbans typically worn by those of the Sikh faith. You can view them at http://www.sikhnet.com/pages/tyingturbans

# History of the Turban and Its Technology

*By SS Ek Ong Kaar Kaur Khalsa*

During Guru Gobind Singh's time, the turban, or "dastar" as it is called in Persian, carried a totally different connotation from a European hat. The turban represented respectability and was a sign of nobility and royalty. At that time, a Mughal aristocrat or a Hindu Rajput could be distinguished by his turban. The Hindu Rajputs were the only Hindus allowed to wear ornate turbans, carry weapons, and keep their mustache and beard. Also at this time, only the Rajputs could have Singh ("lion") or Kaur ("princess") as their second name. Even the Gurus did not have Singh as part of their name, until the Tenth Guru himself gave them that name and took it for himself.

The followers of the Sikh faith did not have the means to display aristocratic attire, nor were they allowed to, even if they did have the means. Doing so was usually equivalent to a death sentence. In this environment,

Guru Gobind Singh decided to turn the tables on the ruling aristocracy by commanding every Sikh to carry a sword, take up the name Singh or Kaur, keep their kesh (hair), and boldly display their turban, without any fear. This effectively made his followers see themselves on a par with the Mughal rulers. The turban is the Guru's gift to us. It is how we crown ourselves as the Singhs and Kaurs who sit on the throne of commitment to our own higher consciousness. For men and women alike, the turban conveys royalty, grace, and uniqueness. It is a signal to others that we live in the image of Infinity and are dedicated to serving all. The turban represents complete commitment.

# Wearing White

Though wearing white (preferably cotton or other natural fabric) clothing is not necessarily part of the Sikh tradition in India, as Western Sikhs who largely came to this path through the practice of Kundalini Yoga and the technology that Yogi Bhajan taught, we usually do wear white turbans and clothing whenever practical. White is universal, in that it reflects all colors, and white light holds the wavelengths of the whole spectrum of colors. So it magnifies the strength of our electromagnetic field, or *aura*, and deflects negativity around us. White also represents purity—of the physical body as well as the consciousness. Notice, if you have a chance, how you feel and what you think when you see someone dressed all in white. Wearing white also makes us more aware and conscious of our actions, because it shows the dirt easily! Natural fabrics are kinder to our electromagnetic fields as well, because they allow unobstructed energy flow. Wearing all white is a technology and an experience that anyone can have. Try it, see how it makes you feel. You may like it!

# Tools to Elevate Our Consciousness

## Banis : Five Daily Prayers

Every day, Sikhs recite five special prayers known as *banis*. These daily *banis* were given to the *Khalsa* by Guru Gobind Singh as tools for people to raise their consciousness and bring balance into their lives. Each *bani* relates to an element (*tattva*), and is usually recited at a specific time of the day. Here are the banis with their corresponding elements:

| | |
|---|---|
| *Japji, Shabd Hazare* | Ether |
| *Jaap Sahib, Tavprasad Swaye* | Air |
| *Anand Sahib* | Fire |
| *Rehiras (includes Bentee Chaupaee)* | Water |
| *Kirtan Sohila* | Earth |

Reciting the *Banis* in *Gurbani* (the sacred language of *Gurmukhi*) gives you a very powerful meditative mind. It brings you the mental and emotional balance required in life. Energy comes to a person from the head, and the head is the distributing center through the spine.

The *Banis* are best recited from the book of daily prayers *(gutkaa* or *nitnem)*. Even though you may have them memorized, you'll be less likely to get distracted and pulled into your own thoughts. For the best effect, a person reads *Gurbani* in the correct harmony and rhythm.

# Power and Effects of the Daily Banis

**Japji Sahib** – connects you with your soul. This is the prayer that begins the Aquarian Sadhana. When your being is endangered, when the radiance of your soul is weak, recite *Japji*. Guru Nanak said that the thirty-eight *pauris* (stanzas) of *Japji* would liberate humanity from the cycles of birth and death. It is said that each of its verses *(pauris)* has additional specific effects and benefits.[36]

**Shabd Hazare** – written by Arjan to his own father, Guru Ram Das, it was the highest love letter ever written. Its gift is that it gives the benefits of reciting a thousand *shabds,* so that one's soul will ultimately merge directly with God. It enables separated ones to come home with grace. Those who recite this shabd will never be separated from their beloved, and will never be separated from the Guru.

**Jaap Sahib** – brings rulership, self-command, and self-grace. It takes away fear and brings vitality, courage, power, strength, and self-esteem. It brings royalty, divinity, bliss, bountifulness, beauty, and grace. The *naad* of *Jaap Sahib* rouses the soul and the self of the Being. ("Sahib" also means grace.) Recite it when your position is endangered, or when your authoritative personality is weak. It will also give you the ability that, no matter what people say, you will automatically be able to compute what they are *actually* saying. Once you are able to recite it correctly, it will give you the *siddhi* (yogic power) that whatever you say must happen (Vakh siddhi). Guru Gobind Singh gave us *Jaap Sahib* so we won't become beggars at anyone's door.

**Tavprasad Swaye** – spoken by Guru Gobind Singh, this is the bani to recite when you are not getting any satisfaction out of life, when life seems to have no juice or flavor.

**Anand Sahib** – Guru Amar Das gave us this Song of Bliss. Mind and body are explained in relation to cosmic divinity. This shabd not only brings bliss, it can make up for deficiencies in the body. It organizes and brings happiness, harmony, and peace. It makes you beautiful, bountiful, and blissful.

A wonderful way for husband and wife to merge together is to recite *Anand Sahib* together, alternating *sutras* (lines). It is said that whoever recites the forty *pauris* of *Anand Sahib* will have endless bliss. Try it yourself and find out!

---

[36] A beautiful special deck of cards, "Guru Nanak's Japji: Song of the Soul" (2005, Sikh Dharma), lists each pauri and its power. They are also listed in the book "Psyche of the Soul" (1993, Hand Made Books, 899 N. Wilmot, Suite C-2, Tucson, AZ 85711), which gives detailed information about the effects and benefits of each of the *pauris* in *Japji.*

**Rehiras Sahib** – You've worked all day, and you're tired; now is the time to recite this *bani*. It adds energy (*raa-hu*) to your being. It brings prosperity, so also recite it when your worldly wealth is endangered. *Rehiras Sahib* helps you when you are physically weak, or weak in money, property, and earthly goods. (In *naad*, *reh* means "live" and *raas* means "commodity," so *Rehiraas* means "living commodity.")

**Bayntee Chaaopaee** is Guru Gobind Singh's personal prayer for protection. It takes care of everything from beginning to end.

**Kirtan Sohila** – is the most harmonious *naad* ever uttered. Recite it at bedtime, just before going to sleep at night. It brings clarity of mind, preserves your night, and brings a beautiful dawn. It prevents nightmares and creates a shield of protection. It multiplies the *aura* to such sensitivity of protection that it eliminates any negativity for miles and miles around you. When you are endangered by any direct or indirect source, and when you want to surround yourself with the protection of the entire magnetic field of the earth, recite *Kirtan Sohila*. At the end of life in this human body, *Kirtan Sohila* is recited to protect the soul on its journey to its True Home with God.

# *Missing Three Days*

Of all the marvelous events in the life of Guru Nanak, perhaps the most outstanding is how he delivered the great epic poem *Japji Sahib*. Here's how it happened:

It was Nanak's habit to bathe in a river every morning before sunrise. One day he walked into the water to take his morning bath (some historians say he went into the woods), and he just disappeared. There was no sign of him. For three days people waited and watched. Finally, when they tearfully assumed he must be dead, he appeared, radiant and shining. With no preamble, he spoke, uttering the immortal words that became the opening phrases of the entire *Siri Guru Granth Sahib*, encapsulating the essence of ultimate Truth. He stated:

EK ONG KAR. "There is One God who created this creation."

Then he said, SAT NAM. "His Identity is Truth." Following that, he described the attributes of the One Creator—as virtues for everyone to develop and practice. Guru Nanak continued speaking, and his words formed a *Mul Mantra* (root sound current).

Later he added forty *pauris* or steps to this *Mul Mantra*, explaining the purpose of life, and the relationship of God to His creatures. This entire composition, in exquisite poetry, is called "*Japji Sahib*"—the Song of the Soul. It is said that the rest of the *Siri Guru Granth Sahib* is a further exposition on the basic Truth that Guru Nanak pronounced on that auspicious day when he emerged from three days of meditation and delivered this gift of divine revelation to the world.

# *The Story of One Grandmother's Nitnem*

At Khalsa Women's Training Camp one summer, Yogi Bhajan told the following story.

"There is a surprising story about my grandmother. She never spoke in a loud voice. I have never seen that woman offending anybody, and I have never seen a single human being offend her. The respect was so great that everyone would settle disputes by Mataji's decision, without going to court.

"Whatever she would say, people would accept it as the truth and nothing but the truth. That reputation and non-offensiveness was built from her perfection of her *Nitnem*, her *sadhana*, and *Gurbani*.

"I am trying to illustrate to you that after a certain age in life, if you do not have nitnem and sadhana, then you will not churn yourself. When milk is churned, it takes a lot of milk to make a little butter. As milk has to be churned to make butter, life has to be churned. Gurbani works to churn the brainwaves through the hypothalamus. You need not be a Sikh. In India, for example, there are a lot of Hindus and Muslims who recite Gurbani. Gurbani is for a person who wants to be graceful, a person who wants to be balanced, and a person who wants to do things by their radiance. A person's presence alone should see the job done."

## Chapter Six

# The Light of the Gurus

✦

Guru Nanak had nine human successors. Nine different men (including one very young boy) to each of whom the same divine light of Truth was transmitted, giving them the ability to inspire and guide their followers to experience the Truth (of God) within themselves as Nanak had done.

Guru Nanak's human successors were from many different walks of life, setting examples to show that everyone has the potential to live as a saint, whether rich or poor, young or old, married or single. Each of the ten Gurus in human form personified certain virtues, and in manifesting these special qualities they became living examples for people in all walks of life to realize they also can experience for themselves the God within themselves.

Here are the main features for which each Guru is remembered:

Guru Nanak – humility

Guru Angad – obedience

Guru Amar Das – equality

Guru Ram Das – service

Guru Arjan – self-sacrifice

Guru Hargobind – justice

Guru Har Rai – mercy

Guru Harkrishan – purity

Guru Tegh Bahadur – tranquility

Guru Gobind Singh – royal courage

And here are some highlights from their lives. For even more detailed biographies, visit www.sikhiwiki.org

# Guru Nanak

## The First Sikh Guru
### (1469–1539)

As was customary in India in the 1400s, an astrologer was called to cast the horoscope for a newborn infant. He amazed everyone by saying, "This is no ordinary child. This infant is a divine incarnation." He predicted that this soul would have a profound influence on the world. The astrologer was definitely right, for the child grew up to be Guru Nanak, the first in the line of Sikh Gurus.

Born in a culture where people lived by the caste system and looked to the priesthood and so-called "holy men" as their connection to God, Nanak and his companion Mardana, who was born a Muslim, traveled on foot over thousands of miles across India and Asia to enlighten people with simple songs of devotion. Everywhere they went, people's hearts were opened and filled with the love of God and humanity.

In addition to being a poet and a singer, Guru Nanak was a great saint, seer, mystic, and prophet. He rejected the notion of divisions between people based on religion. He taught that there is only One Creator who created all of us, so there exists a fundamental brotherhood and sisterhood among all human beings. His simple but profound teachings were firmly rooted in the basic divine identity of all people. When lived with awareness of the Divine Light within everyone, human life becomes a profound experience of love and truth, bringing patience, peace, and contentment. His universal message is as true today as it was then. Listening to his words and songs, we are reminded of who we really are, just as his listeners discovered then.

Guru Nanak achieved enlightenment sometime around the age of 30. After disappearing into a river and meditating in the water for three days, he emerged having had a powerful vision of the nature of reality, divinity, and human existence. He sang that vision in the song known as *Japji Sahib*—the "Song of the Soul." Described in his own words, *Japji Sahib* gives a rare picture of what a Master experienced at the moment of his enlightenment. It became the foundation of a new spiritual tradition.

Guru Nanak traveled extensively. He brought together people from all walks of life, from beggars and thieves to kings and slaves. After his travels, he formed what today we would call a "commune" or "spiritual community" at a small village called Kartarpur (City of God), where he lived as a farmer with his family, working side by side in the fields each day with his students and continuing to teach everyone who came to learn from him.

### *Guru Nanak chooses his successor:*

In Indian culture, sons inherit whatever their father leaves behind. So you might expect that since Guru Nanak had two sons, he would name one of them as his successor, but he didn't. He had specific criteria. He knew the Sikhs needed someone with deep understanding, sincere humility, and faithful commitment to carry on the work Guru Nanak had begun.

Here's how he met his most ardent and faithful devotee.

By the time Nanak was about 51 years old, he was still living at Kartarpur with his wife and sons, still working in the fields every day. Everyone shared in the harvest and ate in the common kitchen. In this communal setting, Guru Nanak wore the simple clothing of an ordinary Punjabi peasant.

One day, he was out in the fields as usual when a man arrived on horseback. Dismounting at a respectful distance, the man humbly announced, "I am Lehna." Guru Nanak replied, "I have been waiting for you—I must pay your debt." (In Punjabi, *lehna* means creditor or debt.)

That's how Lehna's lifetime of service, obedience, and devotion began, which led to his becoming guru Nanak's successor. But I'm getting ahead of my story.

Lehna was the son of a wealthy trader, and he had been an ardent worshipper of the Hindu goddess Durga. While meditating on Durga early one morning, he heard his neighbor Jodha reciting a hymn, which stirred Lehna's soul and opened his heart in a most remarkable way. As soon as dawn broke, he rushed over to ask Jodha where he had learned such divine words. Jodha told him it was a hymn by Guru Nanak. He went on to tell Lehna as much as he knew about this divine teacher who lived in Kartarpur.

This was at the time of year when Lehna customarily led a group of pilgrims to the temple at Jwalamukhi, devoted to the goddess Durga. On the way, Lehna told the others he wanted to stop at Kartarpur, so he could visit Guru Nanak. But the members of the group didn't agree. He was stuck. As the leader, he was supposed to continue the pilgrimage. However, he had such a great longing to meet Guru Nanak that he prayed day and night until one night he was no longer able to resist the magnetic attraction of the Guru's divine light. He just got on his horse and rode. The next morning, he found his Guru working in the fields at Kartarpur.

Without hesitation, without looking back, Lehna began serving in every way possible. He worked in the fields; he served in the kitchen; he sat with the Sikhs joyfully singing Guru Nanak's hymns. He soon went to the Guru and asked to stay with him and to become a Sikh. Guru Nanak told Lehna that before he joined him permanently he should return to his wife and children and settle his household affairs—which he did, making sure everyone was provided for.

# The First Test

On the day Lehna returned to Kartarpur, he was wearing silk clothes that were appropriate for him as the son of a wealthy man. Looking for his beloved Master, he hurried to the fields and found Guru Nanak standing beside three bales of hay that needed to be carried home to feed the cattle. The bales were wet and muddy from rains earlier that day, and the peasants didn't want to carry them. Guru Nanak asked his sons to carry them, but they refused, saying they would send a servant back from the house to do it. Hearing his Master's request, without a moment's hesitation, Lehna picked up the dirty bales and bundling them on top of each other, carried all three of them home.

Of course, his silk clothes were covered with dirt and mud, and Mata Sulakhani, Guru Nanak's wife, was horrified to see a guest in that condition. But Guru Nanak told her, "The load has been carried by the one who was fit to carry it." Furthermore, he told her that it wasn't dirt on his clothes, but saffron. Sure enough, when she looked again, that's what she saw.

# The Second Test

During the winter rains, one of the walls of Guru Nanak's house fell down. He said that he wanted it rebuilt immediately, that very night. His sons asked, "Why not wait until the next morning when it can be easily repaired by the masons?"

Lehna volunteered to do the job immediately. Just as it was finished, all smooth and mortared, Guru Nanak passed by and said, "It's all uneven." Without hesitation, Lehna tore down what he had painstakingly built, and started all over again. Once more when it was done, Guru Nanak looked at it and said he wasn't satisfied with the work. Once again, without complaint, Lehna started from scratch. Guru Nanak's sons watched all this, and told Lehna not to pay any attention to "the crazy old man." Lehna ignored them and continued obeying the Master's wishes. Finally after many attempts, the job was done and met with the Guru's approval.

A teacher has to test a disciple's obedience and ability to surrender. Yogi Bhajan told us, "To be a great leader; you first have to be a great student."

# A New Name

Guru Nanak had observed Lehna's behavior closely for a long time, and one day he placed his hand upon Lehna's head and called him Angad—a "limb" of his own body.

It seemed pretty obvious that Angad would be Guru Nanak's successor, but there was still another test that proved that he was the right choice for this exalted position of leadership and responsibility.

# The Final (and most famous) Test

When Guru Nanak was out walking with his sons and a group of Sikhs one day, they came upon a platform on which there seemed to be a corpse covered with a sheet. Guru Nanak said, "Eat it." Everyone just laughed at this shocking order. Angad said simply, "At which end should I begin, Master?" When the sheet was pulled back, it revealed food spread out on a table. Before eating anything himself, Angad offered food first to Guru Nanak and then the others, saying that he would eat whatever was left over. This principle of first sharing with others is known in Sikh Dharma as *Vand ke chakna.*[37]

---

[37] See page 76

# *Guru Angad Dev*

## *The Second Guru Nanak*
## (1504–1552)

Angad was 25 years old when he became the Second Guru. He went into seclusion to meditate; however, after six months, he was convinced to return to active leadership. As a leader, he set an ideal example , living and serving as Guru Nanak had done.

Guru Angad was very fond of children, organized games for them and even gave out prizes. He took special interest in their education, which undoubtedly led him to work on the *Gurmukhi* script which made Guru Nanak's teachings easily available so even children could read them.

## GURMUKHI: *One of Guru Angad's Most Important and Valuable Contributions*

Before Guru Angad simplified *Gurmukhi* ("from the mouth of the Guru"), only the Brahmins, the priestly class, could read. They were paid by the illiterate to read and perform ceremonies for them. Guru Angad gathered Guru Nanak's hymns, which were in various scripts or had been memorized by some of his disciples, and rewrote them plus his own compositions in *Gurmukhi*, a simple phonetic script. *Gurmukhi* was so easy to read that everyone could learn it. This codified script elevated the lower classes and was a means to directly experience the divine. *Gurmukhi* is and endures today as the "language" in which the entire *Siri Guru Granth Sahib* is written.

# Guru Amar Das

. . . . . . . . . . . . . . . . . . . . . . . . . . . . . . . . . . . . . . . . . . . . . . . . . . .

## The Third Nanak
### (1479–1574)

Amar Das was a Hindu of the Vaishnav faith. He was a sincere seeker of spiritual truth. Every year for twelve years, he bathed in the sacred Ganges River. He also fasted regularly. Despite his earnest religious efforts, he still felt empty inside. During his last pilgrimage to the Ganges, he befriended a monk, and they traveled home together. After several days, the monk asked him, "Who is your guru?" Amar Das had to admit he didn't have one. The Monk was horrified. He said that he had committed a sin by traveling with a man who had no guru, and therefore he would have to return immediately to the Ganges to purify himself! This astonished Amar Das, and set him to thinking that not having a guru, a teacher or personal spiritual guide, might be the cause of his dissatisfaction.

. . . . . . . . . . . . . . . . . . . . . . . . . . . .

*Ed. Note:*

*The Siri Singh Sahib said that a person without a guru is like an orphan.*

. . . . . . . . . . . . . . . . . . . . . . . . . . . .

Amar Das lived near his nephew, who was married to Guru Angad's daughter, Bibi Amro. One early morning a few days after his fruitless pilgrimage to the Ganges, Amar Das heard her reciting Guru Nanak's epic poem, *Japji Sahib*. He was absolutely entranced. He thought it was the most beautiful thing he had ever heard.

For several mornings, Amar Das secretly listened to Bibi Amro reciting *Japji Sahib* and singing *sloks* (stanzas) from *Asa di Var*.[38] The divine words touched his soul deeply. In appreciation and reverence, he bowed to her and humbly asked who had written them. Bibi Amro told him all about Guru Nanak, and explained that her father, Guru Angad, was his successor. Amar Das was so excited, he could hardly wait to meet the great soul who had been chosen to carry the divine light of Guru Nanak. Perhaps this might be the guru he was seeking!

The year was 1540 and Amar Das was 61 years old. When he came into Guru Angad's presence, Amar Das felt such divine bliss filling the emptiness within his soul, that he immediately prostrated himself at the Guru's feet. From that moment on, he devoted his life to serving the Guru.

One of Guru Angad's disciples was having a township built on the banks of the river Beas as a tribute to him in gratitude for helping settle a legal dispute. Some of the man's enemies, however, kept undermining the construction by sneaking in at night and destroying the masonry. Guru Angad sent Amar Das to personally oversee the work. When Goindwal was finished, it contained a gorgeous mansion intended for Guru Angad. However, the Guru directed Amar Das to live there in his place. This he did, moving his entire family to the new township. Still, early every morning Amar Das continued to get water from the river that was now four miles away, and carry it to Guru Angad for his morning bath. He would stay and serve him all day long, only returning to Goindwal at night.

---

[38]  Another beautiful poem by Guru Nanak that is usually recited in the early morning.

# Six Turbans

Every six months, Guru Angad gave *saropas* (scarves of honor) to his devotees for outstanding service. Amar Das had been given six such scarves. He put each one on top of the previous ones, wearing them as turbans on his head. He didn't want to remove any of them, since he felt it would be disrespectful to discard such a gift from his master. Eventually this situation was brought to Guru Angad's attention. He had Amar Das brought to him, and had the turbans removed, revealing sores and scabs—since his head and hair had not been washed in three years! He bathed Amar Das' head, healed him, and blessed him for his deep devotion.

# Becoming The Guru

Amar Das' service, loyalty, and devotion were so outstanding that he was the obvious choice when it came time for Guru Angad to name a successor. As had become the tradition, *Bhai Buddha* was called and told of the decision, and Amar Das was installed as the Third Guru Nanak at the age of 73.

# Jealousy

Dasu and Datu, Guru Angad's sons, were jealous of Amar Das, and resented that their father had not named either of them as his successor. Datu even went so far as to set himself up as Guru in the town of Khadur, but people pretty much ignored him, and continued to go in great numbers to Goindwal to bow at the feet of Guru Amar Das. Datu was so angry that he went to confront Amar Das. He said, "How dare you style yourself as Master? You were just a menial servant in my father's house!" Not content with verbally abusing the Guru, he punctuated his insults with a nasty kick. Guru Amar Das took hold of Datu's foot and massaged it, saying, "Oh, honored sir, pardon me, my old bones must have hurt your tender foot."

# Seclusion

In spite of his well-earned and authentic position of spiritual leadership, Guru Amar Das left Goindwal and went into seclusion in his ancestral village of Basarke, a small village in the Amritsar district of the Punjab. He barricaded himself in a small room and put up a sign on the door saying, "He who opens this door is no Sikh of mine, nor am I his Guru." Many days passed, and his Sikhs, determined to see their Guru, couldn't find him. Wise old Baba Buddha[39] suggested they turn Guru Amar Das' mare loose, and the horse would lead them directly to the Guru. When they got to Guru Amar Das' hut, they saw the warning note on the door. Following Baba Buddha's advice, they broke open the back wall of the hut, and entered that way,

---

[39]  Baba Buddha was a most respected saint. He occupies a unique position in Sikh history. He applied the *tilak* (mark) of guruship to five Gurus, saw seven Gurus, and remained in close association with the first six Sikh Gurus from 1521 to 1628 for over one hundred years.

leaving the door untouched. Baba Buddha urged Guru Amar Das to return, saying, "You have tied us to the hem of your garment. Where should we go now if you are not to show us the way?" Guru Amar Das was deeply touched by this speech, and he went back to Goindwal with them. The hut is now a famous place of pilgrimage. Its wall is still broken.

# Equality

Guru Amar Das said that God rewards patience and the Guru helps those who have endurance. He advocated humility, compassion, and serving people of God. He maintained a free kitchen providing bountiful food, while he himself ate only two very simple meals a day. Guru Amar Das insisted that before anyone could get an audience with him, they must first eat in the free kitchen. People of all castes, peasants and royalty, Hindus and Muslims, all sat together, side by side, in the same *langar* lines.

To carry Guru Nanak's teachings far and wide, Guru Amar Das trained 146 teachers, including fifty-two women, thus adding practical emphasis to Guru Nanak's respect and appreciation for women. These teachers traveled extensively to minister to the spiritual needs of the growing number of the Guru's followers. Furthering the concept of community, Guru Amar Das also established twenty-two centers (*manjis*) presided over by devout Sikhs.

He taught that the pilgrimages, penances, and Hindu rituals that had been appropriate for the three previous Ages[40]—*Sat Yug, Dwarpar Yug*, and *Treta Yug*—were no longer suitable nor effective in this Age, the Kaliyug. The only thing that can earn salvation is meditating on and repeating God's Name.

Guru Amar Das had copies made of the prayers and poems of Guru Nanak and Guru Angad, and then added his own verses. All these divine words of wisdom were read at the many *manjis* he had established all over India.

He denounced *purdah*, the veiling of a woman's face in public, and *sati*, the tradition that expected a widow to burn herself on her husband's funeral pyre, a practice that Guru Nanak himself had condemned.

Guru Amar Das also appealed to the Sikhs to live a family life, what he called *ghrist-mai-udas:* "renunciation in the midst of the world." Or, we might translate it as, "Living in the world but not of it." An ancient analogy of such non-attachment to the world is the pure lotus flower that floats pristine and pure on the surface of the water, yet has its roots in the mud below. Guru Amar Das is the author of this ideal definition of marriage: "They are not husband and wife who merely sit together; rather they are husband and wife who have one soul in two bodies."

---

[40]  See chapter on Aquarian Age/Yugas, page 23

# *Eighty-four Steps at Goindwal*

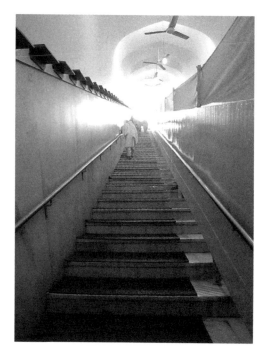

Guru Amar Das decided to build a baoli, an open well with broad steps leading down to the water, to provide a "holy dip" to pilgrims visiting Goindwal en route to the towns of Hardwar, Varnasi, and Kasi. After offering prayers, many devoted Sikhs dug deep enough to reach water, but a large rock blocked any further progress. Guru Amar Das could tell that in order to complete the work, they would have to blast the slab of rock out of the way and risk being drowned. A young man, Manak Chand of Vairowal, volunteered to do the dangerous task. When the slab cracked, he couldn't get out of the way fast enough, and the force of the water was so powerful, he was drowned. His wife wept inconsolably while his mother deeply mourned the loss of her son. Out of pity and compassion, Guru Amar Das called out Manak's name, and it is said that he came back to life.

After the remaining steps were completed, the Guru said that whoever recites *Japji* on each of the eighty-four steps would be freed from the cycle of birth and death. (There are 8.4 million possible life form incarnations for all creatures.)

# Guru Ram Das

# The Fourth Nanak
## (1534–1581)

## Yogi Bhajan's Nighttime Visitor

In 1938, when he was 9 years old, Harbhajan Singh Puri (who grew up to be Yogi Bhajan) was seriously ill with a severe ear infection. Neither his father, Kartar Singh Puri, who was a physician, nor any other doctor and healer that had been consulted, could find a cure. The infection was spreading, and if it reached his brain, he would die.

While he slept, the boy had a visitor—you can call it a dream or a vision, if you wish. Guru Ram Das came to young Harbhajan Singh and told him that he should ask his father to put a little onion juice in his infected ear. The boy told his father, who was willing to try, and sure enough, the treatment worked.

From that time on, Harbhajan Singh considered Guru Ram Das as his special protector, teacher, and guide. 3HO ashrams around the world are named in honor of Guru Ram Das, the Fourth Sikh Guru, the great healer and servant of mankind.

Guru Ram Das was a "Raj Yogi" (*Royal Yogi*). He designed *Harimandir Sahib* (Temple of God), the famous Golden Temple in Amritsar, India. Sikhs all over the world consider it the holiest of holy places. Open to people of all religions, colors, and nationalities, tens of thousands of people visit this sacred shrine daily to be inspired and uplifted by the sound current created by the continuous recitation of the *Siri Guru Granth Sahib*, the *Shabd Guru*, and to sip and dip in the healing waters surrounding the Temple.[41]

Every night for four years, during the time he worked for the Indian Government as a customs officer, after his duties were done, Yogi Bhajan went and washed the floors of the Golden Temple. During those hours he prayed to cleanse and purify himself, and even to lose—or at least not misuse—the yogic powers he had gained. He prayed to Guru Ram Das. He went into the Golden Temple as a yogi and came out a saint. Such is the power and majesty of Guru Ram Das.

## Return Visit to India

Very soon after his move to the United States, Yogi Bhajan became enormously popular. His Kundalini Yoga classes were filled to capacity. He captured the hearts and touched the souls of students who felt from him the universal love that only an enlightened master can share. Many students wanted to go with him when he attended Gurdwara on Sundays. When he went back to India for a visit in 1972, eighty-four yoga students went along with him.

---

41  See Chapter 8 for more about the Golden Temple.

Unfortunately, his huge success in the United States stirred up jealousy and envy among some so-called spiritual people in India, and they betrayed his trust in them. I personally wired to India the money that had been collected to build proper accommodations, showers, toilets, and mattresses. His "hosts" simply took the money without making any arrangements. When the travelers arrived, they found that not even a cot had been prepared for their visit.

Yogi Bhajan had to sleep on the cold hard cement floor. Knowing the group could not stay there without decent housing, he gathered up all the students, and they left for Amritsar. Threatened and harassed, he meditated and prayed, calling on Guru Ram Das for help. Guru Ram Das appeared before him again and this time gave him a special mantra to chant for protection whenever he—or anyone—was in danger:

# *Guru Guru Wahe Guru, Guru Ram Das Guru*

When we call upon Guru Ram Das, we are not calling on a person. We are invoking the enlightened consciousness that this great being embodied, and bringing to ourselves his special divine qualities.

*Ram* is one of the names of God, and *Das* means servant. Guru Ram Das was indeed, a beloved servant of God. He was the fourth in the line of Sikh Gurus, having been appointed by Guru Amar Das, his predecessor, who was, by the way, his father-in-law!

## Orphan Boy

Before he became Guru, Ram Das was known as Jetha, which means "first born." Both his father Haridas and his mother Mata Daya (or Anoop Davi) died when he was only seven years old.

# *A Marriage Made in Heaven — or Outside the Window*

One day as Guru Amar Das and his wife were discussing the need to find a husband for their daughter, Bibi Bani, the Guru looked out the window and saw Jetha on the street selling grams (beans), which was his usual occupation. Guru Amar Das said, "There, that's the kind of honest, hardworking, spiritual man who should marry our daughter." "Well," said someone, "Why not actually ask him, then?" And it was arranged!

Guru Amar Das had already met Jetha when he first came to Goindwal with a group of traveling Sikhs, and the Guru had taken note of the handsome young man's hard work, pleasant manner, and the humble attitude of devotion with which he served wherever and whenever needed, even without being asked.

## Jetha: Ambassador to the Mughal Court

Meanwhile, jealous Hindus brought false accusations to the Mughal Emperor, Akbar, against Guru Amar Das for slandering both the Hindu and Muslim religions. Guru Amar Das sent Jetha, who had become a trusted disciple, to the Mughal court as his representative. When Jetha explained the fundamental teachings of the Sikhs to the Emperor, Akbar was so impressed and convinced of the universality of the Sikhs' faith that he dismissed all the charges.

## Three Sons

**Ed. Note:**

*Jealousy seems to rear its ugly head repeatedly in Sikh history. I suppose that whenever there is great light, it must face an assault by darkness in order to burn more brightly. It often boils down to a false sense of entitlement because of lineage, rather than understanding that in the spiritual realm, values and caliber must take precedence, regardless of lineage.*

In due course, Guru Ram Das was married to Bibi Bani (as a married woman she was called Mata Bani), and they had three sons: Prithi Chand, Mahan Dev, and Arjan Mal (who was destined to become the Fifth Guru, Arjan Dev.)

Arjan Mal was exceptionally devoted to his father, and served him so humbly and consciously that he incurred the jealousy of his oldest brother, Prithi Chand. You can read a famous story of how that jealousy backfired on Prithi Chand in the section called *SHABD HAZARE* on page 109.

# Lord of Miracles

A master of Raj Yoga and famous for his extraordinary gift of healing, Guru Ram Das is known as the "The Lord of Miracles." He is loved and revered as an embodiment of compassion, humility, integrity, and service.

At night, Guru Ram Das used to walk in disguise through the streets of Amritsar and wash the feet of poor weary travelers. They were definitely surprised the next day when they came for an audience with the great Guru, and found him to be the same quiet, humble man who had washed their feet the night before!

Guru Ram Das was intimately involved in establishing the site of the *Harimandir Sahib*, the Golden Temple. The location of the famous "nectar tank" in Amritsar was discovered in a most remarkable way. Here's the story:

# Rajini, The Leper, and The Golden Temple

A wealthy *kardar* (tax-collector) had seven virtuous and beautiful daughters. Rajini was the youngest. Her father provided all of his daughters with graceful luxurious environments, the best teachers to cultivate their talents, and the finest clothing and food. He was very affectionate toward them. He was quite proud of his ability to provide so well for his family, and he constantly reminded them of all the things he had given them. This *kardar* had arranged the marriages of his six eldest daughters to wealthy men of good social standing. Soon, it would be Rajini's turn.

One day, all seven sisters had been walking among the lush gardens on the far side of their father's estate. On their way home, they came across some saints in meditation. Rajini was entranced by the sound of these holy men singing God's praises, and she stayed behind to listen. They sang the words of Guru Nanak:

*Naanak junt upaai kai sunmaalay subhanaah. Jin karatai karanaa keeaa chintaabhi karanee taah.*

"O Nanak, He who created the creatures takes care of them all. The Creator who created the creation, He takes care of it too."

*Ed. Note:*

This is the way I recall Yogi Bhajan telling the story. *"This is a true story known to millions of people. It didn't happen thousands of years ago. It happened only a couple of hundred years ago, and it is verifiable. Each spot where Rajini sat is marked and can still be seen. Villagers still tell her story."*

Rajini was so inspired, she took off all her fine jewelry and gave it to the saints to show her gratitude for this marvelous experience. When she got home, she told her sisters about the wonderful words that had touched her heart and soul. They noticed her jewelry was missing, and they asked her where it was. When her parents heard she had given it to the saints, her father summoned all his daughters and asked them, "Who is it that has given you your food, clothing, and jewelry? Who looks after you and takes care of you?" Rajini's six sisters dutifully answered, "It is you, Papaji, who does all this for us." But Rajini gave a different answer. She said, "It is God who provides and takes care of us, as He does for all of His creatures."

Her father was furious. No matter how he put the question, nor how often, Rajini's answer remained the same. This made him even angrier, and out of his rage and huge ego he told her, "You are ungrateful, and it is time for you to leave my house. I am going to marry you to the next man that passes in front of our window!" As fate—or destiny—would have it, a leper who had been brought to the village to beg for food came in sight just then. Her father demanded that Rajini be married to him at once.

Obedient young Rajini had no choice. Her father had ordered it, and his word was law. So the marriage took place. She had a husband who was a leper, a poor misshapen man who couldn't walk, who couldn't feed himself, and who had open seeping wounds all over his body. After the wedding, the whole family took this leper, put him in a basket, and put the basket on Rajini's head and said, "Here's your dowry, and this is your farewell—never come back to us ever again."

Rajini said, "Can I have ten minutes in our house to say a prayer?"

The father said, "No, cut it short and get out. That's it. You get out of here. I don't want to see you. I am sick and tired of your telling me that I do nothing for you and that 'God does everything.'"

The painful story is that Rajini did say her prayer quickly, and in her prayer she said, "God Almighty I am very grateful to you. I am very blessed that you have given to me the man I deserve. My love for you is eternal and all I ask is that You help me to carry this responsibility with utmost grace."

Rajini took the basket with her husband in it, put it back on her head, and walked out of her parents' home. She walked from village to village, getting some food for herself and her husband.

After walking many miles, Rajini, who was very thirsty, came to a pond where the nectar tank of the Golden Temple of Amritsar is today. At that time it was just a very small pond. Under a *Ber* (Banyan) tree she put down the basket containing her husband, covered him, gave him some water to drink, washed his face, washed his hands and said, "Please be so kind as to stay here. I am going to the nearest village to ask for some food or alms so that we can survive. Be peaceful in this basket." So Rajini left her husband by the bank of the pond and went into town.

As her young husband sat in his basket he saw something very unusual. He saw blackbirds come and dive into the pond, and when they flew out, they had turned from black to white, like little angels. He watched this odd scene for a long time, and then he decided to try something. He shook himself out of the basket and rolled himself right into the pond at the place now called *Dukh Banjhan Ber.* That same tree is still there.

He dipped himself in the water, and within a few moments he found to his amazement that he was totally healed. His leper's sores were gone.

But he had kept one finger out of the water. He reasoned, "If she comes and sees me healed she will not recognize me, then I will be able to show her this finger."

When Rajini returned with food she saw this very handsome young man sitting there and she said, "Where is my husband?"

He said, "I am your husband."

She said, "No, no, that's not true! Have you killed that unfortunate leper just because you want to have me? No way! I am married to him, and I will defend my honor with my life!"

Her husband said, "Calm down, calm down. It really is me. I am the same person. Don't you recognize my clothes?"

She said, "Clothes? You must have stolen his clothes."

He said, "No. I am healed. I went in the pond. Look at my finger. See? Now watch this." He dipped that festering finger in the water, and it came out perfect.

She said, "No, no, no, that can't be! I don't believe it."

He said, "All right then. We cannot agree. I say, 'I am your husband,' and you say, 'I don't believe you.' You say, 'My husband is a leper.' I say, 'I am cured. You saw my finger; it got cured. You don't believe it.' You are just being paranoid. In this town lives the saint, Guru Ram Das, let us both go to him and let him decide."

So they went to Guru Ram Das. The Guru looked at them and said, "Rajini, this man is your husband. For centuries people have been trying to find this particular pond. We have already dug *santhok sar*, the tank of contentment, and now we will call this place *Amritsar*, the tank of nectar." Then Guru Ram Das and the entire *sangat* (congregation) went to the pond where Rajini's husband had been left in the basket and blessed the couple.

Circumstances later compelled Rajini's parents to come there, and seeing the miracle that had happened, they offered all their lands to Guru Ram Das. Rajini and her husband lived and ruled there for some time. It was within that area, then called *Chak Ram Das*, or *Ram Das Pur* (City of Guru Ram Das), that Guru Ram Das laid the foundation for the Golden Temple.

# Baba Siri Chand and Guru Ram Das' Beard

Guru Nanak's son Baba Siri Chand insisted upon being a recluse and living as a renunciate. So, in spite of the boy's great spiritual powers, Guru Nanak did not name him as his successor. He advocated marriage for his Sikhs. He did not believe that you had to be a hermit and turn your back on the world in order to live a spiritual life. Baba Siri Chand became the leader of a sect of ascetic yogis called the Udasis.

By the time Guru Ram Das was installed as the Fourth Guru in 1574, Baba Siri Chand had been the head of the Udasis for many years. He decided to visit the renowned Guru Ram Das, and asked him, "Why do you keep such a long beard?" This was quite rude, but Guru Ram Das understood that Baba Siri Chand might still harbor resentment for not having been given the Guruship. So with true love and compassion (not sarcastically, as I might have done!), Guru Ram Das replied, "To wipe the dust off the feet of holy men like yourself." The Guru then leaned over and proceeded to do just that with his beard. Baba Siri Chand was humbled by Guru Ram Das' response and recognized the divine essence that manifested through him. He reached out and put his arms around the Guru. Baba Siri Chand admitted that he finally understood why his father had not chosen him to be his successor.

# Guru Ram Das Outlines the Daily Practice for All Sikhs

*Bhai Gurdas Bhalia*, the son of Guru Amar Das' younger brother, was a superb poet, fluent in many languages, and an accomplished scholar of comparative religion. Based on his extensive knowledge, he wanted to become a Sikh of the Guru and went to Guru Ram Das to offer his commitment. He received the Guru's blessing and became an outstanding devotee. Soon Guru Ram Das sent him to Agra (future site of the famous Taj Mahal) to inspire the growing congregation there. Guru Ram Das told him to establish the ideal daily practice for all Sikhs. Here are the guidelines the Guru gave:

. . . . . . . . . . . . . . . . . . . . . . . . . . . . . . . . . . . . . . . . . . . . . . . . . . . . . . . . . . . . . . . . . . . . . . . . . .

*One who considers himself to be a Sikh of the True Guru shall rise in the early morning hours and meditate on God.*

*Upon arising early in the morning, he is to bathe and cleanse himself in the pool of nectar.*

*Following the Instructions of the Guru, he chants the Name of the Lord. All his misdeeds and negativity shall be erased.*

*Then, at the rising of the sun, he sings Gurbani, and all through the day, whether sitting or standing, he remembers his True Identity.*

*One who meditates on God with every breath and every morsel of food—that Sikh becomes pleasing to the Guru's Mind.*

*The Guru's Teachings are realized by that person unto whom God is kind and compassionate.*

*Servant Nanak begs for the dust of the feet of that Sikh, who chants the Naam and inspires others to chant it.*

*(Rag Gauri Ki Var: Guru Ram Das)*

. . . . . . . . . . . . . . . . . . . . . . . . . . . . . . . . . . . . . . . . . . . . . . . . . . . . . . . . . . . . . . . . . . . . .

# Sacred Pot Luck: "Dish and Wish"

To celebrate Guru Ram Das' birthday, the Siri Singh Sahib began a custom in America of "Bring a Dish and Make a Wish." It's like a sacred potluck dinner. People prepare food consciously with their own hands and bring it to the Gurdwara along with their personal prayer. Then they place the dish prayerfully before the Guru. All the offerings are later served to everyone as *langar.* "Dish and a Wish" has now become a popular way to celebrate other auspicious occasions.

The spirit of Guru Ram Das lives on in the hearts and souls of devotees all over the world. Anyone can call upon Guru Ram Das with love, and experience his blessing. His presence is real and immediate.

# *Guru Arjan Dev*

## *The Fifth Nanak*
## (1563–1606)

Guru Ram Das had three sons. The child who was to become the Guru was the youngest. Born April 15, 1563, he was named Arjan Mal. Each of the boys had very different dispositions. The eldest, Prithi Chand, was clever in social and worldly affairs. He managed the Guru's household and most efficiently administered the running of the common kitchen. He really wanted to become the next Guru, and he knew that it was service, not lineage, which had earned that position for Guru Angad and Guru Amar Das. He made a conspicuous show of serving his father, but his motives were easily seen by Guru Ram Das.

The second son, Mahadev, was a recluse and, contrary to the Guru's teachings, he adopted the ways of an ascetic. He wasn't interested in becoming the next Guru.

From his earliest childhood, Arjan Mal, the youngest of the three, was serenely tranquil and calmly in tune with the Infinite. One day when he was just a baby, Arjan crawled up on Guru Amar Das' seat and sat there quite contentedly. The Third Guru smiled and said, "(He) will carry the Sikhs across in the ship of the *Nam*."

Hearing this prophecy and worried that it could come true, Prithi Chand kept trying to find ways to disrupt the life of Arjan Mal, but he failed every time.

## *The Greatest Love Poem Ever Written*

When Arjan Mal was in his teens, one of Guru Ram Das' cousins came from Lahore to Amritsar especially to invite the Guru to attend his son's wedding. The Guru said, "I am not able to attend but perhaps I can send one of my sons instead."

When Prithi Chand was asked to attend the wedding, he said, "I have to take care of the collections, and anyway, I hate going to weddings." Actually, he was afraid that if he stayed away from the Guru too long, he might lose his chance to be appointed successor. He figured, "out of sight, out of mind."

Guru Ram Das then turned to Mahadev, the son who spent most of his time meditating. Not unexpectedly, Mahadev refused, saying, "I have no desire to involve myself in worldly affairs."

Finally, the Guru asked Arjan Mal who said, "I only desire to do what you wish." Very pleased with this reply, Guru Ram Das told Arjan to share the Guru's teachings with the Sikhs in Lahore and give any donations to the free kitchen to feed the poor. The last words he said to Arjan were, "Stay in Lahore until I send for you in writing."

Arjan Mal stayed in Lahore after the wedding, and all of his relatives and all the other Sikhs he met there grew very fond of him. Still, every moment he was away, his heart was with his father, Guru Ram Das.

When he expressed his longing to see his father to his new friends, they suggested he write a letter asking to return. Arjan wrote a beautiful verse and sent this letter to his father. When the messenger reached Amritsar, Prithi Chand, suspecting he carried a letter from his brother, told him, "I will take the letter to the Guru myself." Prithi Chand read the letter and realized it was so beautiful that it would surely move the Guru's heart in Arjan's favor. Hiding the letter in his coat, he sent the Sikh back to tell Arjan that the Guru said he should stay in Lahore until sent for. When Arjan received this message, he knew that Prithi Chand, and not his father, had sent it. So he sent a second letter with strict orders that it must be given directly to the Guru.

Again Prithi Chand intercepted the letter, grabbing it out of the messenger's hands. Hiding the letter in his coat, he sent back the same message telling Arjan to remain in Lahore until sent for. When Arjan heard this from the messenger, he wrote a third letter. This time he wrote the number "3" on it. He told the messenger to be on his guard against Prithi Chand and to give the letter only to Guru Ram Das in person. This time, the messenger waited until Prithi left the Guru's court and then quickly found the Guru and gave him Arjan's letter.

When the Guru saw the number "3" on this letter, he knew that he had not received the first two. When the messenger told him what had happened, Guru Ram Das called for Prithi Chand and asked him three times if he knew anything about the other letters. Prithi Chand denied it each time. Of course, the Guru knew better. He told the messenger to go to Prithi Chand's house and bring the coat hanging by the door. When he returned with it, the two missing letters were in the pocket. The Guru confronted Prithi Chand with this evidence and his son's lie was revealed in front of the whole congregation.

Immediately the Guru sent Bhai Buddha to Lahore in a carriage to bring Arjan Mal home. Finally united with his father, Arjan humbly placed his head on Guru Ram Das' chest against his long beard, while the Guru hugged him gently in his arms. The Guru said that since Arjan had written three stanzas, he should now write a fourth and finish the poem.

Upon hearing the final verse, Guru Ram Das said, "The Guruship is passed on because of merit. Only one who is most humble can carry it, therefore I grant it to you." Then according to tradition, the Guru sent for a coconut and five *paise* (coins) and placed them before Arjan. He stood up and, in front of the whole sangat, placed Arjan upon his seat. Bhai Buddha pressed the traditional *tilak* (red mark) on the center of Arjan's forehead as a symbol that the light of Guru Ram Das had now passed to him. Thus Arjan Mal became Guru Arjan Dev, the Fifth Sikh Guru.

The poem that Arjan wrote is called "Shabd Hazare." Guru Ram Das announced that the devotion that inspired it was so great that singing it only once equals the power and benefit of singing a thousand shabds! Whoever recites it will never be separated from the Guru or from those they love.

# SHABD HAZARE

*My mind longs for the Guru's darshan*

*It cries out like the thirsty chatrik bird42 waiting for the rain*

*But the rain does not come.*

*I can find no peace without the darshan of my beloved Guru.*

*O my beloved Guru, my soul longs to serve you and have your darshan,*

*II*

*Your face is so beautiful and hearing your bani brings me deep peace.*

*It has been so long since this chatrik has seen any water.*

*O, my dearest friend, O my beloved Guru.*

*Blessed is the ground beneath your feet.*

*My soul longs to serve my dearest friend, my beloved Guru.*

*III*

*Every moment I am away from you is the whole Kali Yug for me.*

*When will I see you, O my beloved Master?*

*I cannot get through the night without the sight of your Court.*

*I cannot fall asleep.*

*My soul longs to serve at my True Guru's Holy Court.*

*IV*

*I am blessed, for I am with my Saintly Guru.*

*I have found the Eternal God within myself.*

*I will serve you every moment of my life, and never be away from you again.*

*I devote my body and soul to your service.*

*O my Master, slave Nanak lives to serve you.*

Although he was only 18 when he became the fifth Sikh Guru, Arjan possessed deep spiritual understanding and an angelic quality that easily touched the hearts of his devotees. Throughout his entire life, Guru Arjan Dev was always filled with deep inner peace.

---

42  *Chatrik*: A family of songbirds that includes the peafowl, nightingale, cuckoo and kohel. They cannot drink water from a pool, so they sit on their perch and catch raindrops in their beaks.

# Guru Arjan Dev's Service

In the true spirit of "There is no Hindu, nor Muslim..." Guru Arjan Dev with the help of Mian Mir, a Muslim Saint from Lahore, laid the foundation of *Harimandir Sahib*, the present Golden Temple. It has entrances open on all four sides, signifying that all four castes are welcome to enter.

Along with the Golden Temple, the city of Amritsar came into existence. Guru Arjan Dev also created new cities at Kartapur, Tarn Taran—with its magnificent healing tank, and Baoli at Lahore.

# The Birth of the Guru Granth Sahib

The preparation of the Guru Granth Sahib was one of the great achievements of Guru Arjan Dev. He had three goals. First, he intended to preserve the original sacred Hymns composed by the first four Gurus and protect them from being distorted by impostors. Second, he wanted to give the world an everlasting guiding light, a physical and spiritual touchstone. Third and most of all, he wanted to establish the Sikhs as a casteless and secular society. Along with verses composed by the first four Sikh Gurus plus his own, he also included the divinely inspired words of other enlightened men: Sheikh Farid, a Muslim saint; Bhagat Kabir, a Muslim weaver; Bhagat Ravi Das, a shoemaker from Uttar Pradesh; Dhanna, a farmer from Rajastan; Namdev, a calico printer from Maharashtra; Bhikhan, a Sufi saint; Jai Dev, a poet from Bengal; Trilochan, a Brahmin from Maharashtra; Sur Das, a blind poet; Pipa, a king from Uttar Pradesh; and several more, all belonging to different walks of life, sects, and both high and low castes. Guru Arjan Dev himself was a gifted and prolific poet. More than half of the *Siri Guru Granth Sahib* is made up of his writings.

## Dasvandh

Guru Ram Das had introduced the institution of Masands (representatives of the Gurus) who served in different locations. Guru Arjan Dev added the principle of Dasvandh, tithing, the giving of one tenth of every individual's income toward the Guru's *Langar* and for supporting other acts of benevolence to the poor. He told his Sikhs that one tenth of the earnings we receive does not belong to us; it belongs to God—the One who gives us all ten tenths! When we give one-tenth back to Him, all the wealth and prosperity that is ours is revealed to us and is bestowed upon us. If we fail to give God that tenth part, which is rightfully His, it is still due and we may see unexpected expenses. This law of life is a cosmic inevitability.

## Master Musician

Guru Arjan Dev loved music, and was expert in the *Ragas*, traditional Indian musical tonal patterns. When the professional musicians who sang hymns at the Guru's court became egotistically proud of their talents, he introduced the tradition of having the entire *Sangat* sing together, instead of just listening to "performances" by the *Ragis*.

# Events Leading Up to the Martyrdom of
# Guru Arjan Dev

Emperor Akbar was already convinced of the spirituality of the Sikh Gurus. During one of his campaigns, he had come to Goindwal where he ate *langar*, sitting on the floor like everyone else before paying his respects to Guru Amar Das.

A Muslim Pir, the Saint Mian Mir from Lahore, loved and served Guru Arjan Dev and the Sikhs. Mian Mir was very revered by the Emperor Akbar. Consequently, when charges were leveled against Guru Arjan in Akbar's Court by a few impostors (Prithi Chand and his son Meharban) and some jealous Hindu Priests (*Brahmins*), the charges were totally disregarded. The complainants were virtually thrown out of King Akbar's court.

The House of Guru Nanak had gained enormous popularity under the guiding light of Guru Arjan Dev. Both Hindus and Muslims flocked to the Guru to pay homage. The dismay of fanatic Orthodox Muslims at the growing number of Guru Arjan Dev's followers was heightened by the malicious manipulations of Chandu Shah, a Hindu revenue official at the provincial court of the Emperor at Lahore. Chandu Shah had once offered his daughter in marriage to Guru Arjan Dev's only son Hargobind, but the offer had been refused. "Hell hath no fury…"

But Akbar did not reign forever. Emperor Jehangir was of a different caliber. He wrote in his biography, "A Hindu named Arjan lived at Goindwal…simple-minded Hindus and ignorant and foolish Muslims have been persuaded to adopt his ways… this business has been flourishing for three generations. For a long time it has been in my mind to put a stop to this affair and to bring him into the fold of Islam…"

Jehangir summoned Guru Arjan Dev to Lahore. He wanted to have him executed for inciting rebellion. However, on the recommendation of Pir Mian Mir, he commuted the sentence to a fine of 200,000 rupees plus an order to erase a few verses from the Granth Sahib. Guru Arjan Dev would not do it. The Sikhs of Lahore offered to pay the fine, but the Guru refused to let them.

The Guru was imprisoned and brutally tortured. He was made to sit on a heated metal plate, and burning hot sand was poured on his naked body as he sat exposed to the scorching heat of the June sun. Pir Mian Mir asked the Guru why, with his yogic powers, he did not stop the torture.

The Guru told him to close his eyes and watch. Mian Mir saw the Guru sitting on the iron plate pouring the hot sand on himself and also stoking the fire beneath the hot plate. He immediately realized that everything was happening according to God's will and this was the Guru's destiny. The Guru said, "Thy will is sweet to me, O Lord. Nanak craves for the wealth of God's name." The torturers placed Guru Arjan Dev's blistering body in the cold water of the River Ravi. There, his soul was set free.

Guru Arjan Dev was the embodiment of devotion, selfless service, and universal love. In other words, he exemplified spiritual excellence. He contributed deeply to the welfare of the society in which he lived and he stood steadfast for the principles he believed in and for which he gave his life, experiencing the first martyrdom In Sikh history.

Before he died, after serving 25 years as the Fifth Guru, Arjan Dev chose his son Hargobind, to follow in his footsteps and carry the light of Guru Nanak for all humanity.

· · · · · · · · · · · · · · · · · · · · · · · · · · · · · · · · · · · · · · · · · · · · · · · · · · · · · · · · · · · · · · · · · · · · · · · · · · · · · · · · · · · · · · · · · · · · · · · · · · · ·

*NOTE: This chapter is partly based on an article published at www.sikhiwiki.com by: Pritpal Singh Bindra, author and columnist, and winner of the Akali Phoola Singh Book Award 1998.*

· · · · · · · · · · · · · · · · · · · · · · · · · · · · · · · · · · · · · · · · · · · · · · · · · · · · · · · · · · · · · · · · · · · · · · · · · · · · · · · · · · · · · · · · · · · · · · · · · · · ·

# *Guru Hargobind*

## *The Sixth Nanak*
### (1595–1644)

### Setting the Scene

In India endless battles were waged for power and territory. In a culture full of war and revenge, in a climate of fear and hostility, the peacemaker is persecuted.

The martyrdom of Guru Arjan Dev, a man of peace, marked a major turning point in Sikh history. When Guru Arjan Dev's son, Hargobind, became the sixth Nanak, he trained his Sikhs to become warriors so they could defend their rights and the rights of others to live and teach according to their faith.

The advent of the Sikh way of life and the establishment of the Mughal Empire took place at the same time in history. Sikhs were not against Islam. They opposed the feudal and imperial structure that encouraged injustice and exploitation. The scourges of caste divisions, religious discrimination and superstitions made daily life intolerable for ordinary people. The oppressors shielded themselves behind Islam, as well as Hinduism. Guru Hargobind used both the power of prayer and the sword to fight this oppression.

### Death of His Father

Hargobind was only 11 years old when his father, Guru Arjan Dev, was martyred. When he learned of his father's torture and death, he remained calm in his sadness. His father had nobly returned Home to God. He did not grieve because his father had forbidden it. Instead, Hargobind requested the highly respected Baba Buddha to recite the Guru Granth Sahib, and instructed musicians to sing the Guru's hymns.

## *Soldier Saint*

Within ten days, Hargobind was installed as the Guru. Previous Gurus had all worn a woolen string called a *seli* as a sign of the Guruship. When Baba Buddha presented it to Hargobind, the boy proclaimed that he would wear a sword instead. "Sikhs must defend their faith and commit to fight whenever necessary."

Baba Buddha placed a three-foot sword at the Guru's right side. When he went to move it to the customary left side, the Guru asked him to leave it there and put another sword on the other side.

## Miri and Piri

*Ed. Note:*

*This is happening even today in the 21st Century.*

*With the two swords, he demonstrated we must live consciously in the physical world, although the spiritual realm is our real home.*

Guru Hargobind explained the sword on his left, which he called "Miri" (earth), represented earthly power, worldly leadership, and guidance, while the sword on his right was named "Piri" (heaven) and symbolized spiritual authority and power. His purpose was not to mix religion with politics, but to defend the rights of the exploited people against the oppression of the rulers. Bringing religion into politics enabled the Mughals to persecute people. History has many examples of ruling classes oppressing people from behind the shield of religion.

## Martial Arts Training

Guru Hargobind knew there must be a Sikh Army if Sikhs were to survive against their oppressors. He set up training in the military arts: fighting, fencing, hunting, archery, riding, and wrestling. With total devotion, and without pay, young Sikhs flocked to offer their allegiance to him. They were each given a sword and a horse.

He raised the Sikh flag and used large drums (*nagaras*) to get everyone's attention when he made announcements. In 1606, he had the Akal Takhat[43] built in front of *Harimandir Sahib*, the Golden Temple. Seated there, he listened to people's problems and complaints, issued orders, and solved disputes.

## The Guru Visits Emperor Jahangir

Chandu and other enemies of the Guru learned of the Guru's military preparations, and claimed that Guru Hargobind was not only converting Muslims to his faith, he was raising an army to avenge his father's death. With this false rumor, they tried to convince Emperor Jahangir that Hargobind posed a major threat to his kingdom.

The Emperor decided to investigate for himself and invited Guru Hargobind to Delhi. There, the Guru was treated with utmost courtesy. Jahangir discussed religious matters with him and found that the Guru's principles and beliefs posed no threat whatsoever to him or his kingdom.

## The Emperor and the Tiger

In a friendly gesture of hospitality, Jahangir invited Guru Hargobind to go with him on a hunting expedition. As they rode along, a ferocious tiger suddenly appeared out of the thick forest. When the Emperor saw the tiger about to pounce on him, he called out to the Guru to save him. Guru Hargobind, shield and sword in hand, jumped off his horse, ran in front of the Emperor, and with one stroke of his sword killed the tiger. After that Jahangir considered him a true friend, and often invited Guru Hargobind to go hunting with him.

---

[43] See page 147.

In spite of their friendship, the Emperor was jealous of Guru Hargobind's popularity. When he heard that the Guru was called Maharaj ("Greatest King") by his followers, he wasn't really convinced when the Guru told him that God is the only "King of kings." Then an interesting thing happened.

A young grass-cutter, mistaking the Emperor for the Guru, bowed to him, made an offering and pleaded, "O True King, all earthly kings are false. I am a poor Sikh of thine; thy sovereignty is real and potent. Protect me at my last hour and extricate me from hell." The Emperor remembered he hadn't even been able to protect himself from a tiger, so how could he save this man's soul? He returned the grass-cutter's offering and, pointing to Guru Hargobind, said, "He is the True King."

## The Fort at Gwalior

Meanwhile, Chandu continued scheming to undermine the Emperor's relationship with Guru Hargobind. He feared the Guru would try to avenge Guru Arjan Dev's torture and death. At every opportunity, Chandu planted seeds of doubt and jealousy, pointing out the Guru's increasing popularity and power. When Jahangir was ill, Chandu bribed an astrologer to influence the Emperor to send the Guru away on the pretext that in order for the Emperor to recover, a very holy man needed to go to the Fort at Gwalior and pray for his health. The Emperor's ministers pointed out that Guru Hargobind was the obvious choice.

Although Guru Hargobind knew what was going on, he also understood that everything was part of God's plan, so he set off for Gwalior. There he found the prisoners living in terrible conditions without adequate food or clothing. Among the prisoners were *rajas* whose kingdoms and thrones had been taken over by Jahangir. The Guru lived with them, shared his meager rations with them, and comforted them with stories of Guru Nanak and his teachings.

The *rajas* were so grateful they prayed for him and his well being, wishing he could stay with them forever. They became Sikhs.

Meanwhile, Guru Hargobind's mother sent Bhai Buddha to find out why her son had not returned home. Appalled by the conditions in the prison, Bhai Buddha suggested that Guru Hargobind escape. Instead, the Guru wrote to his mother and his Sikhs that he was content living in the Fort where he could meditate without worldly distractions.

Nevertheless, the Sikhs wanted their leader back. They sent representatives to the Emperor asking him to free the Guru. Having had fearful dreams and visions, Jahangir ordered Guru Hargobind's release. However, the Guru refused to leave the prison until all the *rajas* were freed. The Emperor agreed to let them go if the Guru vouched for their loyalty.

It is said that the fifty-two *rajas*, upon hearing they were being released with him, seized the hem of Guru Hargobind's robe and wouldn't let go until he promised them salvation. Sikhs celebrate the holiday *Diwali* in remembrance of this event.

# Guru Hargobind's Greatest Contribution

He turned saints into soldiers and yet remained a man of God. He felt that nonviolence used out of helplessness or fear is cowardice. He made clear that true nonviolence (*ahimsa*) comes from a position of strength and requires standing up to defend the defenseless. He was a strong leader of men and a hero on the battlefield; nevertheless, he was not happy with having to be involved in so much bloodshed. He cared deeply about the spiritual welfare of his people and encouraged them to read from the Guru Granth Sahib, as he did every morning and evening. He named Har Rai, his gentle grandson, as his successor.

# Guru Har Rai

## *The Seventh Nanak*
## (1630–1661)

Har Rai was an extremely sensitive child. The story is told that when he brushed against a rose bush and accidentally knocked some petals to the ground, he wept because he had hurt the bush.

He became the Guru at the age of 14. Honoring his grandfather's wishes, he did not disband the existing army of Sikh Warriors (Saint/ Soldiers) that Guru Hargobind had established. He kept 2,200 mounted soldiers at all times. Although he personally never indulged in any direct political or armed controversy with the Mughal Empire, Guru Har Rai always personally remained a man of peace while encouraging the military spirit of the Sikhs.

He went hunting, not to kill animals, but to care for them in a beautiful zoo he had established at Kiratpur Sahib. He also established an Ayurvedic herbal medicine hospital and research center there.

## *Healing the Enemy*

Dara Shikoh, the eldest son and heir apparent of Shah Jahan[44] became seriously ill, poisoned by his brother Aurangzeb, who aspired to the throne. The best physicians said his only hope for recovery was if he could be given certain medicines they did not have at hand.

Advised that Guru Har Rai had healing skills and these rare medicines, Shah Jahan sent a humble request for treatment for his son. The special medicines were given to the Emperor's messenger with the addition of a pearl that was to be ground up into powder and added to the remedy. The Guru's Sikhs asked Guru Har Rai why he was helping the son of Shah Jahan, an enemy who had quarrelled with both his great-grandfather, Guru Arjan Dev, and his grandfather, Guru Hargobind, and was certainly also his own enemy.

The Guru replied: *"Behold, with one hand man breaks flowers and with one hand offers them, but the flowers perfume both hands alike. The axe cuts the sandal tree, yet the sandal perfumes the axe. We ought, therefore to return good when we are treated badly."*

The medicines saved the life of Dara Shikoh. The Emperor wholeheartedly thanked the Guru and vowed he would never again cause him any annoyance.

---

[44] You remember Shah Jahan, right? He's the Moghul Emperor who built the *Taj Mahal* at Agra in memory of his beloved queen, Mumtaz Mahal.

# Prince Dara Shikoh

As soon as Shah Jahan died, Aurangzeb usurped the throne, chasing away his brother Prince Dara Shikoh. The prince fled the court and took sanctuary with Guru Har Rai. According to the tradition of the Guru's household, Guru Har Rai received Dara Shikoh with great courtesy. Grateful to the Guru for saving his life, the prince confided he was not interested in securing the throne and would rather be left alone for spiritual pursuits. Nevertheless, when he left the Guru's protection, Dara Shikoh was executed, having been falsely accused by his brother Aurangzeb of deviating from Islam.

# Aurangzeb and Baba Ram Rai

Under Aurangzeb, the state turned openly hostile against non-Muslims. Emperor Aurangzeb summoned Guru Har Rai to Delhi under false charges. He let it be known that if the Guru would perform a miracle for him, he would accept him as a man of God. If not, he would punish him as a commoner according to law. Wisely, not trusting the Emperor's motives, Guru Har Rai decided not to go to Delhi. His son Baba Ram Rai insisted they should not offend Aurangzeb and volunteered to go to court to represent the Guru.

Guru Har Rai agreed, but warned Ram Rai not to indulge in miracle-making. Guru Hargobind had particularly forbidden it, and he did not approve of it either. Furthermore, he must not allow the sanctity of the Guru Granth Sahib to be compromised at any cost.

Once Ram Rai was at court, he worked miracles one after another to humor the king. When Aurangzeb expressed his objection to one of Guru Nanak's verses in the Guru Granth Sahib that mentioned Muslims, Ram Rai said the word "Muslim" was a mistake, and he changed it to please the Emperor.

When Guru Har Rai was told what had happened, he excluded Ram Rai from the Sikh *Panth*[45] and refused ever to see him again, though his son begged for forgiveness. Thus Guru Har Rai established the strict policy of never altering the original words in the Guru Granth Sahib.

Because of Ram Rai's disobedience and distortion of the sacred words of the Guru Granth Sahib, Guru Har Rai chose his younger son, five-year-old Har Krishan, as his successor. Shortly before his untimely death at the age of 30, Guru Har Rai had the little boy installed as the Eighth Guru.

---

[45] *Panth:* The entire body of Sikhs.

# Guru Har Krishan

## The Eighth Nanak
### (1656–1664)

Though each of the Gurus was different in personality, appearance, and age, they all shared the necessary virtues of humility, obedience, and loyalty. Thus, despite his young age, Har Krishan was chosen to lead the Sikhs.

## The Bhagavad Gita Test

Pundits (scholars) and other village intellectuals were not happy, to say the least, about having to bow to a little child as their Guru. To test his spiritual authority, they asked Har Krishan to give them a dissertation on the *Bhagavad Gita*.

Har Krishan refused and told them to send for Chhajjoo, a simple water carrier. Chhajjoo was considered to be the "village idiot." He never spoke and people thought he was deaf. Everyone pretty much ignored him. When Chhajjoo was brought before him, Guru Harkrishan touched him and immediately this deaf-mute began to speak, eloquently interpreting the meaning and importance of the famous *Gita*.

> "Those who are destined to lead must first learn to follow."

This story is very important to share with students training to become Kundalini Yoga teachers, some of whom may be a bit insecure about their ability to teach. This story illustrates (in case you missed the point) that God can work through *anyone*. Ego isn't just thinking you're better than other people; ego is also believing that you are not good enough, or unworthy. A good teacher of Kundalini Yoga knows that he or she is just an instrument, and that God and Guru can work through anybody, you just have to show up (and tune in!). That's why we always chant ONG NAMO GURU DEV NAMO at the beginning of each class. This sound current invokes the blessings of the Creator and the Divine Teacher within everyone.

## Guru Harkrishan in Delhi

Ram Rai was furious that his little brother had become the Guru, which he felt was his rightful due. He set himself up in Delhi as the Guru, and appointed corrupt Masands who collected donations for him using threats and blackmail.

When Ram Rai learned that Guru Har Rai had told Har Krishan never to see the Emperor Aurangzeb, he saw an opportunity for revenge, and convinced the Emperor to invite the young new Guru to visit him in

Delhi. If Guru Harkrishan refused the invitation, it would offend the Emperor, and if he did show up, that would offend the Guru's devotees. Fortunately, Raja Jai Singh, who was devoted to the Sikh Gurus, figured that if Guru Harkrishan would at least come to Delhi, that would satisfy the Emperor, and so he urged him to come, with the assurance that he didn't have to actually meet Aurangzeb.

## Smallpox

A smallpox epidemic swept through Delhi, and many people sought Guru Harkrishan's help, as he was known to be a natural healer. Many people were healed in his presence. He met a large number of devotees daily so it is not surprising that he contracted the deadly disease himself. With a raging fever, he asked to be moved from his residence in Delhi to a house on the banks of the river Jumana. Knowing he was dying, he consoled his grief-stricken mother and devotees, reminding them that everything was God's will. He asked them not to mourn. Guru Har Krishan was barely eight years old when he left his body, having endeared himself to everyone with his gentle loving nature, combined with wisdom far beyond his years. The divine light of Guru Nanak shone brightly, if briefly, through this child.

## Naming His Successor, "Baba Bakala"

Before he breathed his last, Guru Har Krishan said that the next Guru would be "Baba Bakala." Everyone there understood that he meant the Guru would be found living in the town of Bakala. And there begins the next story about pretenders to the throne!

# Guru Tegh Bahadur

## The Ninth Nanak
### (1621–1664)

*Ed. Note:*
*Guru Tegh Bahadur's writings form the final portion of the Siri Guru Granth Sahib. Called the sloks, these verses are recited by the whole congregation at the end of every Akhand Path.*

Guru Tegh Bahadur holds a unique place in the history of all religious martyrs, because he didn't sacrifice his life for his own Sikh religion, but for the religious freedom of the Hindus. That story comes later. First, to give you a picture of the kind of man he was, here are some stories about his life.

## Background

When Guru Tegh Bahadur was born, he was named Tyal Mal (master of unattachment). He lived with his father Guru Hargobind and his mother Nanaki in the city of Amritsar, where he studied Sikh scriptures with Bhai Gurdas and learned how to use weapons.

Remember, his father, Guru Hargobind , had been the first Guru to take arms and fight back against the persecution and religious prejudice rampant in the country.

In keeping with the Sikh ethic of earning one's living by honest labor, he was sent to live and work at Ramdas Farm with the revered Baba Buddha who, even though he was then quite old, still labored in the fields every day.

Naturally calm and introspective, when his beloved mentor died in late 1631, Tyal Mal became even more quiet and withdrawn. However, honoring the Sikh ideal of living a family life, he was married to Bibi Gujri in March of 1632. He was 11 years old. Two years later, when Painde Khan and the Moghuls attacked Kartarpur, he fought so bravely and fiercely alongside his father Guru Hargobind, that the Guru praised him for his expert swordsmanship and renamed him "Tegh Bahadur.[46]

## Living in Bakala

As you know, each Guru who followed Guru Nanak named a successor before he died, and in 1644, just before his death, Guru Hargobind entrusted the leadership of the Sikhs to his grandson, Har Rai, who

---

[46]  Tegh Bahadur = Brave wielder of the sword.

became the seventh "Guru Nanak." He knew it wasn't time yet to turn over the Guruship to Tegh Bahadur. Instead, Guru Hargobind told him to take his mother Nanaki and his wife Gujri to the village Bakala, where his maternal grandparents lived. And that is where he was living when Guru Har Krishan died.

As I mentioned in the previous chapter, just before Guru Har Krishan left his body, he subtly revealed the identity of Tegh Bahadur as his successor by indicating where the next Guru could be found, simply by saying, "Guru Baba at Bakala." But of course some of his relatives who were "pretenders to the throne" figured that they could profit from this vague description by going to Bakala and setting themselves up as the next Guru.

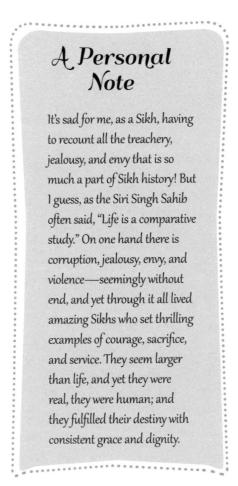

## A Personal Note

It's sad for me, as a Sikh, having to recount all the treachery, jealousy, and envy that is so much a part of Sikh history! But I guess, as the Siri Singh Sahib often said, "Life is a comparative study." On one hand there is corruption, jealousy, envy, and violence—seemingly without end, and yet through it all lived amazing Sikhs who set thrilling examples of courage, sacrifice, and service. They seem larger than life, and yet they were real, they were human; and they fulfilled their destiny with consistent grace and dignity.

## A Merchant Trader Keeps His Promise

A merchant trader named Makhan Shah also went to Bakala to find the Guru in order to honor a pledge he had made to give him five gold coins for rescuing his ship and its valuable cargo from a great storm off the port of Surat. Makhan Shah saw a lot of people in Bakala claiming to be the Guru, but he knew there could only be one True Guru. So he offered two gold coins to each of the false gurus, all of whom were quite happy to receive the money. But when he offered two coins to the genuine Guru, Tegh Bahadur, the Guru said, "Where is the rest of what you promised me?" Then the Guru showed him scars on his shoulder and explained he had gotten them when he was pushing Makhan Shah's ship to the safety of the shore! That was all Makhan Shah needed to hear. He didn't need any other proof. Here, indeed, was the True Guru. He was so excited; he climbed to the roof of a house and shouted at the top of his lungs, "I have found the Guru! I have found the Guru!" He told the story of the miraculous rescue of his ship and soon all the sincere devotees recognized that Guru Tegh Bahadur was definitely the rightful leader of the Sikhs. (This was not good news for the false gurus, who wouldn't be receiving any more gifts and offerings!)

## The Jealous Nephew

Guru Tegh Bahadur had an older brother, Baba Gurditta. Baba Gurditta's older son, Dhir Mall, was one of those who had hoped to be accepted as the Guru, and so when he learned that Tegh Bahadur had been acknowledged as the true Guru, he figured the only way he could take over the leadership (for the money and power it would bring) would be to have Tegh Bahadur killed. He led a party for that purpose to the Guru's home, and one of the men actually shot Guru Tegh Bahadur. The bullet grazed the Guru's forehead and drew some blood, then glanced off his skull sideways but left him otherwise unharmed.

The thieves stole whatever they could lay their hands on, including a volume of sacred writings. Shortly thereafter, Makhan Shah arrived at the scene, and when he found out what had happened, he took a group of men and went to Dhir Mall's camp where he captured him along with one accomplice (the rest of the scoundrels had run away). He retrieved all the loot they had taken from the Guru's house, tied up the men there, and brought them barefooted into Guru Tegh Bahadur's presence. Observing his nephew's pathetic condition, Guru Tegh Bahadur instructed Makhan Shah to release the prisoners and give them everything they had stolen from him. He said the money and goods they had stolen had brought them nothing but suffering and disgrace, and so it should stay with them—except, of course, for the volume of sacred Sikh writings—that, he knew, belonged in the Guru's house.

## Locked Out of the Golden Temple

Guru Tegh Bahadur headed for Amritsar in order to stop Har Ji (Prithi Chand's[47] grandson) who was having his own poetry recited in *Harimandir Sahib*, the Golden Temple, claiming it to be the Guru's words. When Har Ji learned that Guru Tegh Bahadur was coming toward the *Harimandir Sahib*, he got the *masands* (caretakers, sevadars, and tax collectors) to lock the visitors' entrance. So, though Guru Tegh Bahadur and his party were able to dip in the sacred pool, they couldn't get inside the Temple. The Guru would not let Makhan Shah and his men force their way in, as they wanted to do, so they left. The Guru said, "Because of their greed, these people are already dead. There is no use in punishing the dead. In their greed to get the money offered in worship, they have lost all sense of devotion, chastity, virtue, and knowledge, so they cannot be prevented from doing misdeeds."

---

[47]  Remember Prithi Chand? He's the older brother who stole the beautiful devotional letters Guru Arjan Dev had written to their father, Guru Ram Das.

## Anandpur Sahib

The city we now know as Anandpur Sahib (City of Bliss) was originally a village called Makhowal in Kehloor State. Its ruler, Raja Tara Chand, had just died, and his widow, the *rani* (queen), asked Guru Tegh Bahadur to come there for her husband's last rites. Her family had great reverence and respect for the Gurus, especially after the famous event in which Guru Hargobind (the Sixth Guru) had secured the release of her husband, the late Raja Tara Chand, from Gwalior Fort where he was one of the fifty-two rajas imprisoned there by King Jahangir. After the funeral, Guru Tegh Bahadur spoke with the queen and expressed his wish to buy the village called Makhowal, which she now owned. He recognized that it was a natural fort, easy to defend and strategically located in the mountains. He knew that soon there would be attacks on the Sikhs by the Emperor Aurangzeb, the king of Delhi, and he wanted to be prepared.

The queen offered to give him Makhowal as a gift, but he insisted on paying for it, and for five hundred rupees the village ownership was transferred into his name.

# *Architect and City Planner*

Guru Tegh Bahadur personally drew up a map planning the layout of the new city, indicating the location of the streets, bazaars, and residential areas, keeping in mind the need for defense in case of attack. It wasn't until his son Gobind Rai came to live there that the name of the city was changed to Anandpur.

The foundation stone was laid by Baba Gurditta, the grandson of Baba Buddha, on June 19, 1665.

. . . . . . . . . . . . . . . . . . . . . . . . . . . . . . . . . . . . . . . . . . . . . . . . . . . . . . . . . . . . . . . . . . . .

**Ed. Note**:

*June 19th is meaningful to me, because that's my birth date, except, of course, I was born in 1929, 264 years later. When I visited India in 1974, Anandpur Sahib was the place I loved the most, the place where I felt most "at home." Standing inside the Fort at Anandpur Sahib, I could almost hear the echo of the hoof beats that resounded there so many lifetimes ago. I recall that the Gurdwara there served delicious **langar**, including blue cornmeal chapattis. When they brought out the display of Guru Gobind Singh's weapons in the Gurdwara, it was awesome! I remember thinking how strange it was that I, who had been brought up as a pacifist, could experience such a thrill at seeing these magnificent huge **shasters**. They seemed to be sizzling with megawatts of energy and power.*

. . . . . . . . . . . . . . . . . . . . . . . . . . . . . . . . . . . . . . . . . . . . . . . . . . . . . . . . . . . . . . . . . . . .

## No Smoking

Guru Tegh Bahadur was adamant about prohibiting Sikhs from smoking, going so far as to tell them they should not even cultivate tobacco as a crop. Smoking had become very widespread at the time, even among the poor, because it was both relaxing and cheap. Because of the increasing demand due to its extremely addictive qualities, raising it for sale was an easy way to make money. The Guru is quoted as saying (to a Sikh farmer in the village Barna), "My dear Sikh, give up the use of tobacco. Do not even touch it. If you bring it in the house, not only disease but poverty also will harass you."[48] Unlike other substances such as cannabis ("weed" or marijuana) or alcohol, which have a profound effect on the mind, tobacco was not forbidden by other religions, only by the Sikhs. Nowadays we know that smoking causes cancer—and even second-hand smoke is deadly. Yet millions of people all over the world continue to smoke! Isn't human nature interesting?

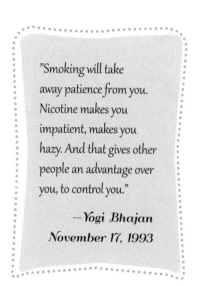

"Smoking will take away patience from you. Nicotine makes you impatient, makes you hazy. And that gives other people an advantage over you, to control you."

—*Yogi Bhajan*
*November 17, 1993*

# *Rituals*

It was customary for the Brahmins (Hindu high-priest caste) to recommend that people bathe in certain rivers to cleanse themselves of past misdeeds. Guru Tegh Bahadur debunked this superstition, saying, among other things, "…You may wash a bitter melon with water as many times as you like from the outside, but the inner bitterness like poison remains in it. In the same way the curse of bad deeds remains with you even after bathing in the river." He added that it could even be harmful if people get the mistaken idea that they were free to do wrong again if they could simply come back and wash all their "sins" away.

This reminds me of a young woman who worked for my mother when I was a child. She would go out and drink heavily, and God knows what else, on Saturday nights, and then go to confession on Sunday morning. Of course, when the next weekend came around, it was a repeat performance.

The Guru explained that it is only by remembering and experiencing our True Identity at each moment that we become free. Sikh Dharma has a different concept of "sin." A sin is simply any act that makes us feel alone and separate from the One in everyone.

---

[48] *Bedtime Stories – 4 Guru Tegh Bahadur Ji*, by Santokh Singh Jagdev, page 34.

# Meeting with Aurangzeb

The powerful king of Delhi sent for Guru Tegh Bahadur, expecting him to perform some miracles for him. He'd seen what Ram Rai could do, and he was eager to meet the renowned Ninth Guru. When he arrived, Guru Tegh Bahadur was greeted with due reverence and respect. He was given a seat near Aurangzeb, who said, "Show me a miracle." The Guru said that to perform a miracle is just the ego, and that all things happen naturally in the Will of God. A better miracle, he said, would be for the great King, who had been given the sovereignty of all India, to treat all religions as equal, and to rule with justice, humility, and kindness. Guru Tegh Bahadur used an analogy to make his point. He spoke of the country's subjects being like cows and goats. "The more you nourish them, the more milk they will yield. The King, who harasses his subjects, destroys himself. There is no place in the house of God for those who indulge in oppression and tyranny."

Aurangzeb expressed his wish that Islam become the one and only religion in India, as that was his way of eliminating religious conflicts. He told the Guru if he would personally embrace Islam, Aurangzeb would make him the supreme religious head of the country and provide him with a very large estate.

Guru Tegh Bahadur politely told him that religion is only a method to experience God, and that everyone should be able to choose their own path, saying, "Faith is the privilege of every individual."[49] He said that conflicts arise out of jealousy, and what the Emperor was offering meant nothing to him. Aurangzeb was so impressed with the humility and spiritual awareness of Guru Tegh Bahadur that he issued orders that the Guru could travel wherever he wished and teach freely, without interference from the government.

## Agra and Mai Bhago

Mai Bhago is one of the women in Sikh history especially remembered for the power of her devotion. Old and frail, she lived in the time of Guru Tegh Bahadur, and from what she had heard of him, she was filled with love and devotion, constantly visualizing him in her mind. She made a robe for him out of cloth she had spun with her own hands while she prayed to see him in person.

Drawn by the strength of her pure prayer, Guru Tegh Bahadur appeared at her door while he was en route to the eastern provinces. Her devotion was so powerful, he stayed in her home where she served him with great joy for over a month.

## Ascetic Versus Householder

In Agra, Guru Tegh Bahadur continued to reinforce the teachings of Guru Nanak. He spoke with a man who was planning to leave his wife and three children to live as a renunciate, a lifestyle ascetics claimed as necessary to "find God." The Guru explained this was an error in thinking. Living in the world and having a family and wealth doesn't stand in the way of God-realization; attachment to people and things is the problem. He asked him, "If you abandon your work and your family, who is going to feed you? You'll still be hungry and end up begging for food from householders! It's greed that needs to be renounced, not wealth."

---

49  *Bedtime Stories – 4 Guru Tegh Bahadur Ji*, page 40.

# Banaras

The sacred river Ganges flows through the city of Banaras. To this day, pilgrims come from all over to bathe in its holy waters. Guru Tegh Bahadur stopped Bhai Jwehri Maal who had been a follower of Guru Nanak's teachings for a long time, as he was heading for the river. The Guru explained to him that the place of pilgrimage for Sikhs is being in the company of holy people and not a river or any other physical location. He dramatically demonstrated that the Ganges flows to the Sikhs, Sikhs don't need to go to the Ganges, by having Bhai Jwehri Maal pick up the rocks under their feet where, sure enough, clear water was flowing.

It is even said that in Banaras, a leper came into Guru Tegh Bahadur's presence, praying to be healed. The Guru instructed the musicians to sing a particular verse, and the leper's pain disappeared.

Over and over he reminded people that it is by reciting the Name of God that the "five thieves—lust, anger, greed, pride, and attachment—can be overcome." The Siri Singh Sahib referred to these five as sisters who are so fond of each other that if you let one in the door, the others follow!

Guru Tegh Bahadur educated scholarly Pundits that it is not reading scriptures that is valuable, but rather living your daily life according to the wisdom they contain.

# Sacred Thread and Barley Balls

As Nanak had refused to wear the cotton thread that was a rite of passage for Hindu boys, Guru Tegh Bahadur did not take part in a ceremony of his time. He pointed out the futility of *Pind*, the custom of throwing balls made of barley flour into water after the Brahmins perform a ritual over them (for which, of course, the priests get paid). These balls supposedly reach the person's dead ancestors (after being eaten by the creatures in the water). You can imagine what Guru Tegh Bahadur said about this practice, especially after the Brahmins admitted that if people didn't follow these customs, the priests would have no source of income.

# Judge Not

The Guru reminded people not to judge others. He taught that the reality of a person is often different from what appears on the surface. He simply would not tolerate gossip or worthless talk. When some Sikhs complained to the Guru about the irresponsible behavior of a Sikh known as Bhai Jagta, Guru Tegh Bahadur advised they should spend a day with Bhai Jagta. They found out for themselves how wrong they had been in their criticism.

This reminds me of the Native American saying, "Never judge a man until you've walked a mile in his moccasins." In Patanjali's sutras[50] it is pointed out in the list of *niyams* and *yams* (the ethical precepts that are the basic attitudes and actions that someone aspiring to reach God Consciousness must practice) that unless one is a parent or teacher, it is none of our business what anyone else is doing or not doing in their private life. And never to gossip! Oh, how eager we are to tell tales about other people! Even if the stories are true, by gossiping we are adding to our own *karma*!

---

[50]   *How to Know God: The Yoga Aphorisms of Patanjali*, Vedanta Press (translated by Christopher Isherwood and Swami Prabhavananda).

## DIVINE UNION
### by Guru Tegh Bahadur

*SORATH, NINTH MEHL:*

*That man, who in the midst of pain, does not feel pain, who is not affected by
pleasure, affection or fear, and who looks alike upon gold and dust; who is not
swayed by either slander or praise, nor affected by greed, attachment or pride; who
remains unaffected by joy and sorrow, honor and dishonor; who renounces all hopes
and desires and remains free from desire in the world; who is not touched by sexual
desire or anger, within his heart, God dwells. That man, blessed by Guru's Grace,
understands this way. O Nanak, he merges with the Lord of the Universe,
like water with water.*

(Siri Guru Granth Sahib, page 633)

# Martyrdom of the Ninth Guru

So, how did Guru Tegh Bahadur come to be a martyr?

The persecution of the Hindus escalated under Emperor Aurangzeb's cruel reign. Somehow it was suggested that if a very holy man would convert to Islam, then all the Hindus would follow suit. Guru Tegh Bahadur mentioned this proposed "bargain" one day in the presence of his thirteen-year-old son, Gobind Rai, who immediately said, "Father, you are the most holy man I know. You should go and plead for the Hindus, and when you refuse to be converted, he will leave them in peace."

## The Fateful Meeting

Guru Tegh Bahadur knew immediately that this was what he must do. Knowing full well what would happen, he went to the Court and met with the Emperor. Once again, Aurangzeb asked him to perform a miracle, and once again the Guru refused. He also adamantly refused to renounce his faith and even when threatened with death, he held fast. He was duly beheaded -- in public. A note was found on his body that read, "I gave my head, but not my faith."

# Guru Gobind Singh

## The Tenth Nanak
### (1666–1708)

*"Only when all other means have failed is it then righteous to take up the sword."*

*(Guru Gobind Singh)*

Guru Gobind Singh, the Tenth Guru, was an outstanding example of the Sikh ideal of the "Soldier-Saint." A courageous warrior, he was also an inspired poet, and a prolific writer. He is remembered as a valiant defender of the poor, the meek and the oppressed masses of India. In times of battle, Guru Gobind Singh always shot arrows with solid gold tips. That way, if an enemy was killed, the man's family would be able to pay for a good funeral and take care of themselves, and if the enemy soldier was injured, that gold could be used to pay for medicine for him and food to feed his family.

Gobind Rai, the young son of Guru Tegh Bahadur, became the Tenth Guru on November 11, 1675, at the age of 13. He was the last of the Sikh Gurus in human form, because before his death, with his Khalsa name of Guru Gobind Singh, he installed the *Siri Guru Granth Sahib* as the next and perpetual Guru forever.

The Tenth Guru molded Sikh Dharma into its present form with the formation of the *Khalsa* in 1699, and finished compiling the Guru Granth Sahib, which some consider his greatest achievement. It is said that after the martyrdom of Guru Tegh Bahadur, Gobind Rai declared that he would create such a spiritual family (*Panth*) that it would challenge the tyrant rulers in every walk of life to restore justice, equality, and peace for all of mankind. As a prophet, Guru Gobind Singh is unique. His teachings are very scientific and timeless. Unlike some other prophets, he never called himself God or the *only* son of God or the messenger of God. Instead he said that all people are the sons and daughters of God, sharing His Kingdom equally. For himself he used the word "slave" (*banda*), which means servant of God.

*"Those who call me God will fall into the deep pit of hell. Regard me as one of His slaves and have no doubt whatever about it. I am a servant of the Supreme Being; and I have come to behold the wonderful drama of life."*

By the orders of the Mughal Emperor, Nawab Wazir Khan, in 1705, Guru Gobind Singh's two youngest sons, Baba Zorawar Singh ji and Baba Fateh Singh Ji, were martyred by being sealed alive in a brick wall. His two eldest sons, Baba Ajit Singh and Baba Jujar Singh were killed during the prolonged siege of Anandpur that same year. Guru Gobind Singh himself was assassinated three years later by Wazir Khan.

Guru Gobind Singh understood that he had to be the last in the line of the human Gurus, and that henceforth, the light of the Guruship would be invested in the sacred volume known as the *Siri Guru Granth Sahib*. From then on, no Sikh would bow before any man as Guru, but bow only to the Word of God, as embodied in the *Siri Guru Granth Sahib*. Thus, the *Siri Guru Granth Sahib* became once and for all time the revered living Guru of all Sikhs, beyond all personality and human identity.

The Tenth Guru consciously broke the ancient tradition of title by lineage and instituted the reality of legacy.

On October 20, 1708, Guru Gobind Singh, having consciously witnessed the sacrifice of the lives of all his four sons, handed over the sacred legacy of the Guruship to the Shabd Guru, embodied in the *Siri Guru Granth Sahib*.

When he last spoke to his assembled Sikhs, Guru Gobind Singh said,

"As ordained by the One Eternal, a new way of life is promoted. All the Sikhs are asked to accept the Holy Granth as the Guru. Guru Granth should be accepted as the living Guru. Those who wish to meet God, will find Him in the Word."

The unique beauty of this is that the Siri Guru Granth Granth Sahib can neither be altered nor can it be changed in any way. It is a touchstone for all humanity that exists beyond the limitations of time and space, now and in the future.

# Queen Victoria[51] and the Pipal Tree Prophesy

Guru Gobind Singh traveled extensively. Fortunately, a written record of his travels was kept in a small book called *Sakhi Pothi*.[52] A man named Attar Singh made a translation of this historic manuscript, and presented it to Queen Victoria at a ceremony that was held to solemnize her sovereignty over Punjab.

This Sakhi Pothi tells the story of the finding of a very significant Pipal Tree (fig tree). It happened in the year 1704 and was recorded in 1714 or 1715. It is said that when Queen Victoria read the story, two paragraphs in particular caught her attention.

The story she read goes like this:

Guru Gobind Singh was traveling through a district of East Punjab. He decided to camp for a night near a village called Soheva. Next to Guru Gobind Singh's tent was a large Jand tree (Banyan). He told one of his Sikhs to climb up to the top of the big tree and look for a Pipal tree. The man reported back that he saw no Pipal tree in the area. The Guru told him to go look again, and to look more closely this time. This time, nestled within the giant gnarled roots of the old Jand tree, the soldier found a tiny Pipal tree sapling growing.

Guru Gobind Singh said, "Though it does not normally grow in desert areas, this particular Pipal tree will grow into a very large tree. It will grow as big as the Jand tree itself. In fact, it will actually tower over the

[51] The information about the Pipal Tree was extracted and adapted from *Sikh Predictions* by Surindar Singh Kohli.
[52] *Sakhi Pothi* was written by an Udasee yogi (a disciple of Baba Siri Chand, the ascetic yogi son of Guru Nanak). Not much else is known about the writer.

whole Jand tree. When this happens my *Khalsa* will spread into the four corners of the world and the sovereignty of Delhi will be the first prize that will fall into their laps. When the Pipal tree will spread over the Jand tree, then the spirit of the order of the *Khalsa*, which I have enshrined under the command of God Almighty, shall start to work to set up a world-society, which will last for five thousand years. That divine society will enjoy peace and affluence."

When Queen Victoria read these words, knowing there was something mystical behind the invincibility of the Sikh soldiers, she wrote to the Governor General at Calcutta, "Please go and find the village called Soheva, and see if there is a Pipal tree growing in a Jand tree there. Please report back to me the size of Pipal and Jand trees."

It took a couple of months, but finally the reply came back: "Yes, it is there. It is now about four and half yards lower than the Jand tree."

Then she referred the matter to the Royal Botanical Professor, who told her, "Your Majesty, the Pipal tree grows very slowly and it will take the Pipal tree at least one hundred years to grow to the same height as the Jand tree." This put Queen Victoria's mind at rest, and she slept peacefully that night—because as far as she was concerned, the slow rate of growth of the Pipal tree guaranteed one hundred years of uninterrupted British rule in India!

The late Kapur Singh, who passed away in 1986, wrote:

. . . . . . . . . . . . . . . . . . . . . . . . . . . . . . . . . . . . . . . . . . . . . . . . . . . . . . . . . . . . . . . . . . . . . . . . . . .

*"During those days I was a British Officer in one of the districts of the Punjab—about sixty miles from Soheva. I was aware of this story, and the official report sent from India in 1858. In 1942, I made arrangements to travel on horseback to see this tree. It was about two and half yards lower than the highest pinnacle of the Jand tree.*

*"Since 1942 I have not been there, but now I am told that the Sikhs who were expelled from Pakistan areas (during the partition of India in 1946) have settled in those arid areas and have built a magnificent Gurdwara in that place."*

. . . . . . . . . . . . . . . . . . . . . . . . . . . . . . . . . . . . . . . . . . . . . . . . . . . . . . . . . . . . . . . . . . . . . . . . . . .

A student of folklore, who visited the location in August, 1990 writes:

. . . . . . . . . . . . . . . . . . . . . . . . . . . . . . . . . . . . . . . . . . . . . . . . . . . . . . . . . . . . . . . . . . . . . . . . . . .

*"I stayed there for two nights. It is very difficult to see any visible Jand tree at all within the outgrown Pipal tree. During my discussion with a sadhu,*[53] *I found out a number of interesting things. He told me, 'A small branch of the Jand tree still exists, and it is only about nine inches in size. It will be completely eaten up by the Pipal tree by the turn of the century (the year 2001.)'"*

. . . . . . . . . . . . . . . . . . . . . . . . . . . . . . . . . . . . . . . . . . . . . . . . . . . . . . . . . . . . . . . . . . . . . . . . . . .

---

[53] *Sadhu:* A renunciate holy man.

# Chapter Seven

# *Personal Stories Along the Path*

✦

## *My Journey on the Sikh Path*

*By Sat Daya Singh Khalsa*

I began my journey along the Sikh path when my old lifestyle stopped bringing me joy and forward movement. People often asked why I "converted" to the Sikh way of life. I do not look it as a conversion as much as an upgrade. Both the world and my place in it had changed, and my old habits and ways of thinking were producing stagnation and unhappiness. It was as if I was using DOS, and upgraded to Mac OS/X.

I do not feel like I adopted a new religion. I was raised in a very religious household. The cornerstone of my birth religion was the infallible belief that one man was the sole representative of God on earth. If one did not accept this as true, one was denying God. Other religions that I have studied rested on similar premises. I found it difficult to accept that God would disenfranchise anyone who did not have access to these particular teachings.

My definition of religion was a thought system that claims a unique ability to channel God's truth. Sikhs do not see the world in such limited terms. They see God's presence in all of creation. They recognize that God reaches out to every single person on the planet, that every single person is a part of God. I was touched by the Sikhs' compassion for the entire world and for everyone's unique expressions of God. I felt at home in the refusal to negate teachings from other traditions.

Initially I thought I would stop at these very basic truths of the Sikh path. But there was something deeper that was moving me forward along the path.

My first experience with a Sikh (besides play dates with a Sikh pre-school friend when I was three years old) was at a yoga class. The room was full with upwards of a hundred people. The teacher walked in through the back of the class wearing full white *bana*, and I was immediately struck by the power that the woman carried.

In the next few weeks my lifestyle became progressively less fulfilling. I had bottomed out. I realized that I needed an overhaul, and I decided to take an intensive three-week Kundalini Yoga teacher training course. The course instructors were Sikhs. I distinctly remember them walking by me during our early morning sadhana meditations. Their mere presence seemed to diminish my worries and sorrows.

After this teacher training, I began to explore the Sikh lifestyle and history. I never had any decisive moments when I made a decision to become a Sikh. I never had an internal debate on whether to stop cutting my hair, to stop drinking alcohol, or to begin covering my head. I would reach points where the answers to the questions of my identity became obvious. I felt powerful and fulfilled as I gradually adopted the lifestyle.

Initially, I did have concerns about how society would view my appearance. The turban and beard were not looked on favorably in the post-9/11 world. What would my family and friends think? These concerns diminished as I walked down the path. The image and form of a Sikh has been blessed with a power. Negativity cannot enter its space. I am sure that I receive strange looks, but those negative projections cannot enter my space.

The existentialist philosopher Søren Kierkegaard spoke of how the true Christian should imagine that he or she is the only Christian on the planet, and be content in that. While I receive much love and support from my Sikh *sangat* (community), I feel so strong in my identity as a Sikh that I could exist if I were the only Sikh on earth. One *shabd* (holy hymn) we sing says, *"Khalsa mayro Sat Guru poora."* This loosely translates as: *"Khalsa* (the form of purity) is my true way from darkness to light."

People sometimes ask whether I feel as though I am conforming. They assume that I am not free to choose my physical appearance, and that I must be similarly limited in other aspects of my life. Actually, I find the opposite to be true. When I had no structure or discipline in my life, I felt like a boat drifting on the sea. With no constants I could not move myself in the direction in which I wanted to head. With a set discipline and practice, I feel liberated.

Those on the spiritual path are walking up a mountain that has true peace as its summit. There are many different paths up the mountain. There have been holy men who have carved definite paths that, when one follows them, will increase one's chances of a successful journey to the summit. If one does not commit to one path, if one continuously walks a bit on one path before jumping to another path, then one can only progress so much.

I am blessed to have been presented with such a clear trail.

* * *

*Sat Daya Singh lives in Los Angeles with his wife Akal Kaur. An avid hiker, he has hiked the entire Appalachian Trail and has trekked extensively in the Andes and Himalayas. He works at the Writers Guild of America West.*

# Born in India and Raised in North America
· · · · · · · · · · · · · · · · · · · · · · · · · · · · · · · · · · · · · · · · · · · · · · · · · · · · · · · · · · · · · · · ·

*By Harjinder Ruby Kaur Khalsa*

My education as a child, as a young adult, and into my adulthood has been spiritually eclectic.

I was born in the Punjab region of Northern India into a traditional Indian Sikh family. Both of my parents were from Sikh families that date back for hundreds of years. In 1969, when I was five years old, my family and I moved from India to Canada.

That is when everything changed for me. We lived in a predominantly Christian neighborhood, and all our Caucasian neighbors did not know anything about Indians or Sikhs. My classmates could not even pronounce my name, and instead of being called Harjinder, which means "the life or manifestation of God as a human being," I was called "Hairy Ginger." It was just simpler for me to survive in my new environment by insisting that everyone call me Ruby, which was my family's nickname for me. Since they really had no idea who we were or what Sikhs represented, we found that if we wanted someone to know more about us, we had to tell them. This was somewhat daunting because contrary to life in our Indian homeland, there were simply no other Sikhs around to whom we could point as examples of our lifestyle.

In fact, believe it or not, in those days there were not even any *Gurdwaras* within several hundred miles of where we lived. When the first provisional *Gurdwara* in a school in Toronto was established, my parents drove my brother and me two and a half hours to get there and two and a half hours to get back. Yes, five hours in a car just to go to *Gurdwara*. And, during the snowy Canadian winter, it took us four to five hours one way. At that time, though, I thought of the trip as a great adventure. Now, as I look back, I realize that the effort my parents extended was motivated by their desire to give us an education about our heritage, culture, legacy, and most importantly, to instill in us the sacred teachings of the Gurus. It was a profound learning experience.

This desire of my parents for us to learn was further exercised when they sent my older brother and me to Catholic Sunday school. Yes, a little Sikh girl was "religiously" taken to Catholic Sunday school to learn. For me, going to a Catholic Sunday school was just another place of God where we socialized with other children and learned about God and God's will. Being from a Sikh family, I had always been trained that "God is One"—*"Ek Ong Kar."* So, we never thought that there was anything weird or wrong with this. Since God is One, it really didn't matter to us who was teaching us about God. The important thing was that we were learning about God.

Coming from this background, it is not surprising that I continued attending the places of worship of many religions. Between the ages of 12 and 16, I used to actually make my friends and neighbors take me to their different Christian denominational churches, including a Jehovah Witness Kingdom Hall, as well as to Muslim mosques, and Jewish synagogues. Furthermore, I felt a compelling urge to learn about the teaching of many faiths. I always had a thirst to learn the words of God as they were spoken in different religions. I would pick up books on theology and read them with the same interest that others would read novels. This continued during my studies at the university level, where I minored in Comparative Religious Studies.

Throughout my teenage years and as a student at the University—quite surprisingly and unexpectedly, even to me—I found that the more I learned about other faiths, the more I cherished being a Sikh. Wow, what an epiphany!

I realized over and over how the Guru's words are all-encompassing. *Hukams* gave me advice that I needed about myself, my friends, family, and even foes. I found the Guru's words to be timeless. They meant something to me when I was five, at 15, and even now as I am 45.

Additionally, I know that the words of the Gurus will have meaning for me in the future and will continue to inspire me to be the best person I can be. Listening to the Guru's teachings, I am ever a student and will remain one till the day I die. The reason is simple; there will always be more for me to learn. I am simply and gratefully a human being, and I will always be a Sikh (student).

It is my Sikh beliefs that have allowed me to be a student of God's word as spoken in many religious teachings. Interestingly, in the process of learning as much as I could about so many religions and faiths, I experienced an immeasurable and constantly growing love and respect for my own Sikh faith and for the vast, all-inclusive teachings of the Gurus emerging from deep within me.

When I look back, I revere my parents' wisdom and can't help but laugh at the road I traveled to come full circle. I am blessed that my parents encouraged us to be Sikhs; yet they never forced us, and in fact, taught us to learn about and respect other faiths, cultures, and ways of life. Thankfully, we were taught to live simply by the words of the Gurus. *Wahe Guru!*

. . . . . . . . . . . . . . . . . . . . . . . . . . . . . . . . . . . . . . . . . . . . . . . . . . . . . . . . . . . . . . . . . . . . . . .

*Indian by birth, Ruby Khalsa is a certified Level One Kundalini Yoga Teacher, who lives in Española, New Mexico, with her husband, a Sikh born in the United States, Siri Mukhta Singh Khalsa.*

. . . . . . . . . . . . . . . . . . . . . . . . . . . . . . . . . . . . . . . . . . . . . . . . . . . . . . . . . . . . . . . . . . . . . . .

# Destined to Stay

· · · · · · · · · · · · · · · · · · · · · · · · · · · · · · · · · · · · · · · · · · · · · · · · · · · · · · · · · · · · · · · · · · · · · · · · · ·

*By MSS Sada Sat Singh Khalsa*

My first encounter with the Guru (in this lifetime) was in February 1973.

I was living at Ahimsa Ashram in Washington, D.C. doing Teacher Training. In those days, Teacher Training in Washington meant teaching the morning Kundalini Yoga class and then going to the restaurant, The Golden Temple Conscious Cookery, to wash dishes and scrub pots and pans until midnight, then go home, get up for sadhana and repeat the process day after day.

I was in this 40-day program because the teacher and Ashram director at Panj Pyare Ashram in Baltimore, where I had been living, suddenly just disappeared. He was with us for an evening meditation and then didn't show up for sadhana the next morning, and that was that. We found out later that he actually went off and joined the Merchant Marines, but that's another story.

Lehri Singh, the Ashram Director and the Eastern Regional Director in Washington D.C., asked me to come to Washington for Teacher Training so I could return to Baltimore to be the new Ashram Director, but the Guru, whom I had not yet met, had other plans for me.

I arrived in Washington, very excited to begin the Teacher Training program. It was a bit of a letdown when I found that my main teacher was going to be two very large pot sinks, a dishwashing machine, and thousands of plates, pots, and pans to wash daily. As Lehri told me, "You already know everything you need to know about Kundalini Yoga, we just want to see if you can keep up." Having just been in the Army, including being a cadet at West Point, I was eager for a challenge and determined to show that I could certainly keep up.

In D.C. at that time, we were also being introduced to the *Siri Guru Granth Sahib* and to Sikh Dharma, so we had begun doing *Akhand Paths* in the Ashram. In those days, we were pretty innocent and uneducated about the Guru. What we lacked in knowledge and experience, we made up in raw devotion…and it was raw. We didn't have a Gurdwara, so we did the *Akhand Path* in a corner of the sadhana room/yoga room/ dining room. There were two rules: 1) Keep your head covered, and 2) Don't stop reading until someone comes to relieve you. Also, don't fall asleep.

With our long workdays and too little sleep, the biggest challenge was staying awake. If you stopped reading, you slept. So you did whatever you needed to do to just keep reading—stand, walk, shout, sing, do frog pose holding the Guru… just keep reading, don't fall asleep, and don't stop until someone comes to relieve you. That was it, plain and simple.

But, sometimes in the "busy-ness" of the restaurant someone might forget their time slot and not show up. That was the one unknown about reading… you just never knew if or when the next reader would show up. Of course, it was an unforgivable act to not show up, so there was a strong commitment and a whole lot of judgment about anyone who didn't show up or forgot their time slot.

After being at the Ashram for about a month, I decided to give this *Akhand Path* thing a try. Also, it sounded like a good break from washing dishes, so I signed up. My dishwashing partner was a little skeptical and worried as in, "What if your relief doesn't show up, and then I'm stuck here alone. I don't like this." I assured him that all would be fine and, "Hey, if no one comes, there's this big bell there that I can ring if I need relief, and there are always people at the Ashram, so someone will come to relieve me—don't worry."

Then, a funny thing happened on my walk from the restaurant to the Ashram. I realized I had had enough of washing dishes… thirty days was long enough, and after a good dose of negativity, *Shakti Pad* or whatever, I figured that this Teacher Training was just a clever way to get cheap devoted labor for the restaurant. (We worked in exchange for Teacher Training.) So I decided to pack my bags and head back to Baltimore.

But, I had committed to read in the *Akhand Path*, and there was that stigma about not showing up, plus I had that military training commitment thing, so I knew I couldn't just not show up. I went down to the basement to the single men's quarters known as the "Nanak Room," and I packed my stuff, which in those days took about five minutes, and went upstairs to read from the Guru. After my hour, the allotted time, the strangest thing happened—no one showed up. Okay, I thought, they'll be here in a few minutes… no problem. But after ten minutes, no one had come.

I started ringing the bell. It was a Saturday afternoon so there were a lot of people coming and going, but still no one came to relieve me. I heard a few comments like, "Keep up… we'll find out who is supposed to be here and go get them." This gave me some hope, but still no one came. So, I began ringing the bell louder and louder and reading as loud as I could to try and get as much attention as possible, but still nobody responded. And now as I'm ringing, I'm noticing people are leaving… to me it looks like a mass exodus from the ashram, and I'm thinking, "They don't want to get stuck here either." In the meantime, I just go on ringing and reading and singing, and two hours go by, and no one shows up.

Now the Ashram is empty, and I can only think, there will be no relief. I'm going to go on reading forever! So, I kept up. Every time someone would come into the Ashram, I'd start ringing the bell, reading at the top of my lungs but no one would come. Two hours became three, and then three became four. After four hours had passed, an interesting thing happened… I got into it. I felt as though I could read forever—which was good, because at that point, I didn't think anyone was ever coming. The four hours then became five, and as the sixth hour arrived, finally someone came. I was relieved! Free at last! But, free to do what?

My bags were packed, and I was ready to go, but all I could think was… okay, already, I got the message! I'll stick around. So, I unpacked, which again took only five minutes, and I made my way back to the restaurant walking on a cloud, to be greeted by a loud chorus of, "Where have you been! We thought you'd never show… get back to work! We need clean dishes!!!"

I could only smile. I had decided to stay. So I rolled up my sleeves and was back at it. I never did return to Baltimore. Those six hours with the Guru put my life in a whole new direction, but as they say, that's another story….

. . . . . . . . . . . . . . . . . . . . . . . . . . . . . . . . . . . . . . . . . . . . . . . . . . . . . . . . . . . . . . . . . . . . . . . . . . . . . . . .

*Sada Sat Singh and his wife, Sada Sat Kaur now live at Yoga Borgo di Guru Ram Das, in the grace and warmth of beautiful Umbria, Italy, where they teach and run a Kundalini Yoga center. Sadasat Kaur has made several wonderful mantra CDs featuring her lovely heart-warming voice.*

. . . . . . . . . . . . . . . . . . . . . . . . . . . . . . . . . . . . . . . . . . . . . . . . . . . . . . . . . . . . . . . . . . . . . . . . . . . . . . . .

# *The First Bhai Sahib of Sikh Dharma: Dayal Singh*

### *By MSS Shakti Parwha Kaur Khalsa*

In August of 1604, when the *Adi Granth*, then known as the *Pothi Sahib*, was installed at *Harimandir Sahib*, the Golden Temple, Guru Arjan Dev, who had compiled this sacred gift to humanity, instructed that, unlike the Hindu Scriptures, anyone of any caste, creed, or gender could read from these Holy pages. When Guru Gobind Singh installed the *Siri Guru Granth Sahib* as his official successor, to be revered as the living Guru, he said, *"He who would wish to see the Guru, let him come and see the Granth. He who would wish to speak to the Guru, let him read and reflect upon what says the Granth. He who would wish to hear the Guru's word, he should with all his heart read the Granth."*

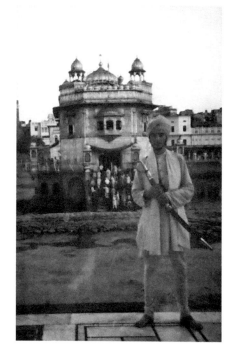

Over 200 years later and 8,000 miles away in Los Angeles, California, a 15-year-old American boy would rediscover his soul's connection with the Guru. The catalyst for this awakening was a talk by the Siri Singh Sahib, Harbhajan Singh Khalsa Yogiji, then known as Yogi Bhajan, who came to Dale Sklar's school one morning in 1970 and spoke about Sikh Dharma, about God and Guru.

This young boy not only began reading from the Granth with all his heart, he taught himself how to read it in *Gurmukhi*. Then he taught other Americans so that they, too, could experience the blessing of the Guru's original words for themselves. I met Dale Sklar when he was 15. He was a student at the school where Yogi Bhajan had gone to give a talk. Yogiji's words had a profound effect on the boy, who soon moved into Adi Shakti Ashram in West Hollywood to be near Guru Ram Das Ashram, and the man he recognized immediately as his Teacher.

Dale took to Sikh Dharma like a duck to water. Dale became "Dayal," which means "kindness." He came to all of the Yogi Bhajan's classes, and incorporated into his life everything he learned. Whatever Yogi Bhajan taught, Dayal put into practice.

His reverence for the Guru, his humility, and good humor—he never had a negative word to say about anybody—made him stand out among all the students.

In 1971, Dayal went to India specifically to do seva at the Golden Temple. He washed the marble floors every night, as he knew Yogi Bhajan had done for four years. On his first trip to India he ate nothing but the *langar* at the *Harimandir Sahib*, and drank the sacred milk/water, which was used to wash the floors of the Golden Temple, a seva he joyfully performed every morning while he was there.

His devotion, seva, and humility, along with the sheer joy he radiated in sharing his love of the Guru, were so contagious and so outstanding that when he came back from India, the Siri Singh Sahib gave him a title and an official position in Sikh Dharma. He appointed him the first Bhai Sahib (Chief Minister) of the Sikh Dharma of the Western Hemisphere.

Bhai Sahib Dayal Singh taught himself to read *Gurmukhi* and then taught others. He took care of the Gurdwara at Guru Ram Das Estate on Preuss Road every day. Without a car, he would walk the five miles from Adi Shakti ashram in West Hollywood twice a day every day to perform the *Prakash* (installing the *Siri Guru Granth Sahib*—literally "waking the Guru") every morning and return in the evening to put the Guru to bed, the ceremony known as *Sukhasan*, covering the Guru for the night. He taught me how to wrap and unwrap the *ramalas*, the decorative cloths that cover the Guru. He taught me which mantras to chant while taking care of the Guru. Always carefully washing his hands before entering the little Gurdwara at the back of the Estate, he would wrap his sleeve around his hand so that his clean hand wouldn't touch the doorknob before he bowed before his beloved Guru. When he turned the pages, he did so carefully, using both hands with a gentle, loving touch.

Bhai Sahib Dayal Singh was beloved by all. He was the epitome of reverence and devotion, yet he was never "holier than thou." He was cheerful and kind to everyone. He never said a bad word about anybody, and I don't think anyone had a bad word to say about him. He was surely a saint. His patience was amazing. The example Bhai Sahib Dayal Singh set in his short life has inspired thousands of others to walk this path.

Once, after a dinner party at Guru Ram Das Estate, Bhai Sahib and I were alone in the dining room when he said to me, "Shakti Ji, you're always telling people what to do, and what they are doing wrong (which was definitely the case in those days!), why don't you ever say anything to me?" I had to reply, "Because there's nothing wrong with you." It was the truth. He was always striving to improve himself.

# SPIRITUAL NAMES

You may have noticed that although many of us Sikhs are Westerners, our names are often not the usual variety you might expect to find in Western countries. We have adopted (often legally) spiritual names that remind us of our destiny as spiritual beings on this planet.

Every soul comes into each lifetime with a particular focus and ability, and a specific destiny to fulfill. Yogi Bhajan used his very developed intuition and a system of numerology (using your birth date) to find the "soul" name. He said that when you meditate on your spiritual name, and deeply understand it, you will know all that you need to know to fulfill your destiny in this lifetime.

A spiritual name becomes almost a personal mantra or hukam that both consciously and subconsciously reminds us of our true identity. When you think about it, our names are probably one of the things we hear and speak the most often in our lives. Now that you have read about the technology of *shabd* and sound current, you can understand how this might work even if we don't know the meaning of the words. Of course, if we do know the meaning of our names, the effect of repeating them often is enhanced, just as knowing the meaning of *Gurbani* enhances the experience of reciting it.

Before the Siri Singh Sahib died, he trained his Chief of Staff, Nirinjan Kaur, in the system he used to determine spiritual names. If you are interested in receiving a spiritual name, you can request it at http://spiritualnames.3ho.org/

Chapter Eight

# *The Guru's Door*

☬

## INVINCIBLE COURAGE AND LEARNING TO BOW

You don't have to think of yourself as a Sikh, just as a seeker, to integrate and complete your daily sadhana practice by participating in a *Gurdwara* (literally the "Gate of the Guru," where everybody can enter). The sacred Golden Temple in Amritsar, the *Harimandir Sahib*, was purposely built with doors open to all four winds, signifying that people of all kinds and all castes, from all directions, were welcome.

The term "Gurdwara" is used to describe the building—or place—where the Guru is installed. Some buildings are elaborate, or individuals may set up a special room as a Gurdwara in their own homes. Gurdwara also refers to what happens, or the worship service that takes place.

On special occasions and Sundays, a big Gurdwara service starts around 10 a.m. until noon, after which *Guru ka langar* is served. Langar is a traditional meal to which everyone is welcome. We have neighbors here in Los Angeles who come on Sundays just in time to have langar! Traditionally, people sit on the floor in long rows, while servers bring steaming buckets of rice, *daal* (beans), and *subzee* (vegetables), while others pass out *chapattis*, the wheat flat bread. Sometimes we have corn tortillas, enchiladas, and salad! If it is someone's birthday, of course there's cake or cookies.

Whatever the food, the important thing is that it is prepared with care and devotion, in a prayerful consciousness. A plate of food is placed before the Guru during the Gurdwara service to be infused with the sacred vibrations. Similarly, the *prashad* has been present during the *kirtan* and *Anand Sahib* (singing of the "Song of Bliss.")

These are not "rituals" done as rote, but are a technology imbued with a sacred reality. For example, when we bow before the Guru with deep humility and devotion, any prayer we offer at that time, as we "offer our head," is most effective. Actually, all we can really offer the Guru, who needs nothing, is all our problems, so when we bow, we can feel free to offer all our worries and concerns to the Guru!

# Saropa: Gift of Honor

When Sikhs want to honor someone, the tradition is to give a gift during a Gurdwara service. This gift is called a *saropa*. It is a token of esteem and appreciation, but a *saropa* is more than just a symbol. It carries the blessings of the entire congregation. A saropa can be in the form of a *mala* (prayer beads) or a piece of jewelry sucwh as a turban pin, perhaps even a *kirpan*, but most often it is a simple piece of cloth, a white or orange scarf or shawl that is put around the recipient's neck and shoulders in much the same way as a lei is presented in Hawaii. The presentation is, of course, accompanied by enthusiastic shouts of *Bole So Nihal –Sat Siri Akal!*[54] The Siri Singh Sahib explained the meaning of this "robe of honor" as follows:

. . . . . . . . . . . . . . . . . . . . . . . . . . . . . . . . . . . . . . . . . . . . . . . . . . . . . . . . . . . . . . . . .

*"Let me tell you about the saropa, why we give it, and what the tradition of it is. With the Saropa, we honor a man from head to toe. Sometimes it's a piece of cloth. But you know, whenever you are in difficulty, if you take that piece of cloth and put it around your neck and you pray, all the mega-vibration, which everybody has prayed for you with it, that can never be disconnected. So saropa is not just a piece of cloth. It's not just a matter of honor. It's a strength, which will always live if you take care of it. Sometimes you bring a saropa from Harimandir Sahib[55], and if you put it on your head, you think it is your head cover. No, it covers you all the way.*

*Karamee avai kopara nadaree mokh duaar...*

*(Your karmas will all be covered, and the door of freedom will open.)*
*(Japji Sahib, Pauri 4)*

*"Whenever you put that saropa around your neck and you do prayer, all those who are there shall ever be bound down to pray with you. It's never just a piece of cloth. It is the psyche and the magnetic field, and it's the person and the magnitude. It's a question of enforcing impact and projecting balance so that the mental*

---

[54] "Those who answer this call will be blessed: Truth is great and undying."

[55] At Harimandir Sahib, after devotees bow to the Guru they are given orange-colored turban-sized pieces of cloth.

*negativity may be wiped out. And it is from that tradition, that people have been given saropas from the Guru's house, because that seals the psyche of all humans and their spirit and their power of prayer together.*

*"... Therefore please understand what these saropas are all about. [When] we put [the saropa] around our neck, and we ask for a prayer, the Sangat[56] of that day and its seven generations, from angelic to the present, and angelic to the future to come shall pray with that man. That's the power of Saropa."*

Gurdwara is open to everyone, regardless of age, race, religion, or gender. If you do not have access to a Gurdwara, with the Shabd Guru, you can actually take a hukam online at www.Sikhnet.com  Finally, say a prayer and sing the "Longtime Sunshine" song.

# The Golden Temple

### By MSS Guruka Singh Khalsa

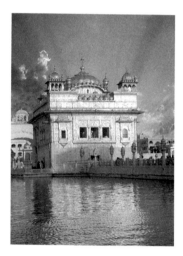

The Golden Temple is the energetic and spiritual center of the Sikh path. It was built in what is now the city of Amritsar in the state of Punjab in northern India during the time of Guru Ram Das and Guru Arjan, the fourth and fifth Sikh Gurus. It was built on the site of an ancient pond known to have miraculous healing powers long before the temple was built. Many stories both past and contemporary have been told of amazing healing that has occurred when devotees come for a "sip and a dip" in the *sarovar,* or "nectar tank," which surrounds the temple itself. The Siri Singh Sahib, Yogi Bhajan, told us many times of the four years he spent doing *seva* (selfless service) washing the floors of the Golden Temple in order to clear any remaining *karmas,* drop negative ego, and expand completely into the master and spiritual teacher he was to become.

Water is like a battery for sound. It holds the patterns of vibrations. You may have seen Dr. Masaru Emoto's work about this very thing at http://hado.net/ and in his well-known book, *"Hidden Messages In Water."*[57] It's quite fascinating and helps explain the amazing phenomenon of what people experience at the Golden Temple. The vibrational quality of water is the basis for the *Amrit Sanchar* (Amrit ceremony[58]) and for the nectar tank at the Golden Temple.

The temple itself is quite small (only 40.5 feet long on each side), and sits in the center of a pool of water called the *Sarovar,* which appears black in satellite photos. All around the perimeter of the *sarovar* is a white

---

56  Congregation
57  Atria Publishing (September 20, 2005), ISBN 978-0743289801.
58  See page 168

marble walkway. A 200-foot long causeway, known as the *Darshan Dhoori*, connects the temple to the walkway (*Perkarma)*, which surrounds the pool.

The Golden Temple has four doors, one on each side, which are "open to all four winds," signifying that people of all kinds, creeds, and walks of life from all directions on the earth are equally welcome to enter.

The Golden Temple complex in Amritsar is a giant generator that produces a huge amount of powerful, clear blue light that cleanses the entire planet.

This is an Aquarian Age temple—sitting on the Earth and rooted in the Cosmos—upon entering which, you instantly experience physical spaces that have been constructed to correspond to your own exact spiritual dimensions. Within it, you sense your own natural, healthy human radiance awakening. When you are there, you understand that the temple actually comes to gracefully live inside you throughout the day—like a best friend—wherever you may be on the earth, for the temple is indeed a mirror. Your inner body temple and this physical outer temple perfectly reflect each other and are contained within each other.

The architectural details are as beautiful as the larger dimensions of this structure, which has been completely built according to the *Vastu Shastra* (the Vedic science of living structure, a spiritual, architectural technology known to the sages thousands of years ago).

Every day, tens of thousands of people walk around the Perkarma, always moving in a clockwise direction. The sound current of the Shabd Guru is constantly being generated within the temple itself, and the temple is coated with a layer of copper covered in gold (a great conductor).

Just as an electrical generator rotates a coil within a magnetic field, the electromagnetic fields of the people walking around the walkway, always moving in the same direction, create a continuously moving magnetic field, which amplifies the sound current within the temple, which is then focused by the structure itself. This creates a powerful beam of light that penetrates the axis of the temple and, in fact, the earth itself. Sitting like a crown on the "head" of Mother Earth, it is like a huge etheric cleanser for the planet. …

. . . . . . . . . . . . . . . . . . . . . . . . . . . . . . . . . . . . . . . . . . . . . . . . . . . . . . . . . . . . . . . . . . . . . . . . . . . . . .

*You will understand that the Golden Temple or Harimandir Sahib, which you call it, is God's temple. It has nothing to do with any politics whatsoever... not at all. It is built in a very unique square pattern.*

*There is a main artery of the Earth's psyche, it is called the "ray of light." It covers the earth just as you might knit a sheet in its longitude and latitude, warp and woof, and it crosses itself many times. It fills the whole atmosphere up from the horizon in all time zones in a diagonal pattern.*

*All temples are built on high places. This is the only temple which is built on the lowest point of the city. Around it is the city of Amritsar. The psyche of the air is filled with prana. You cannot leap down and then get up. Do you understand the biorhythm of the life? The energy circles around it, and the reflection of the sun in the water and the power of the psyche of the gold and the marble which represents the Sun and the Moon in one realm which exists in the center of this whole tank, which you call the sarovar. And it purifies itself by the pranic energy. If you have the eye to see it, then you'll see the very rain of life dropping... a rain of pranas dropping and playing and merging with it."*

*Yogi Bhajan, June 6, 1997*

. . . . . . . . . . . . . . . . . . . . . . . . . . . . . . . . . . . . . . . . . . . . . . . . . . . . . . . . . . . . . . . . . . . . . . . . . . . . . .

# The Akal Takhat

### By MSS Guruka Singh Khalsa

Have you noticed that when you enter a public building or a private home, you can feel the energy associated with it? Every physical structure has its own vibratory frequency. Think of entering a monastery or a dance club. Quite a difference! Each structure holds vibrations within it that can be felt by anyone who is sensitive. The Akal Takhat (the Throne of the Eternal) is a beautiful white marble building located in the Golden Temple complex in Amritsar. But it has always been much more than an imposing physical

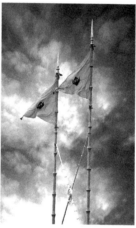

structure. Initially built in 1606 by Guru Hargobind, the Sixth Guru, it has its own powerful, living spiritual identity. As the seat of spiritual sovereignty for all Sikhs, it is a holy place.

In front of the Akal Takhat fly two flags on tall flagpoles. They are called "Miri" and "Piri." Miri means earthly and Piri means spiritual. They signify the balance of earth and ether—matter and spirit—in awakened consciousness. I always say that a Sikh has his head in the stars and his feet on the earth, sees the One in everyone, and remembers his own zip code.

*"Akal Takhat is not what you think. Akal Takhat is not the bricks, the marble, the cement, the house. Akal Takhat is the very creative Infinity and honor of a Sikh. It's not a person. It's not a place, it's not a project. So this concept was given, and this concept demolished death and that made the Sikh deathless."*

*Siri Singh Sahib Ji (Feb 6, 1997)*

## HISTORICAL NOTE:

# Operation Blue Star

On June 6, 1984, the sacred Golden Temple complex was attacked by the Indian army in a planned military maneuver known as "Operation Blue Star." Military tanks stormed the Golden Temple, and literally thousands of Sikhs were killed.

The Indian Army did much more than just damage the outer façade of the Akal Takhat; they destroyed its sanctity. It was blasted with heavy artillery and reduced to rubble, destroying not just the structure, but also all the precious historic artifacts housed within. Although the government later offered to rebuild the Akal Takhat, the Sikhs refused and rebuilt the entire structure themselves entirely by volunteer effort.

When the Siri Singh Sahib spoke on July 1, 1984, about the desecration of the Akal Takhat, he came from a place of cosmic understanding. He wanted to share with us his awareness that the Akal Takhat martyred itself in order to awaken a sleeping spiritual nation.

# Awakening Through Sacrifice: The Akal Takhat

### By Siri Singh Sahib, Bhai Sahib Harbhajan Singh Khalsa Yogiji July 1, 1984, Espanola, New Mexico

*This is the greatest sacrifice that has been made in the history of our lives. The Akal Takhat has offered itself as a sacrifice. To understand this, you have to believe in the identity of the Akal Takhat.*

*Guru Arjan gave the sacrifice; we became victorious. Guru Tegh Bahadur gave the sacrifice; we became victorious. Guru Gobind Singh and his entire family gave the sacrifice, and we became victorious. Today our Akal Takhat has given the sacrifice; we shall not lose!... The Akal Takhat has sacrificed itself to awaken the Khalsa (all people of pure consciousness).*

*... This greatest sacrifice, under the Will of God, has been made to save the planet, to save the humanity, to bring peace and to point us away from destruction.*

### Ed. Note:

*If you have read this far, you will remember the references to events in the history of the evolution of Sikh Dharma, which included the martyrdoms of Guru Arjan Dev and Guru Tegh Bahadur, and the sacrifice of Guru Gobind Singh and his four sons.*

*The Siri Singh Sahib saw and understood the living spiritual identity of the Akal Takhat, whereas most people only saw it as a building, albeit an important one. He also was seeing its martyrdom as a clarion call from the Guru, designed to awaken many Sikhs who needed to return to living as Khalsa: with purity, innocence and courage, as taught by the Gurus and exemplified by Guru Gobind Singh.*

# Sounds of Gurdwara

## Wahe Guru Ji Ka Khalsa, Wahe Guru Ji Ki Fateh!

**Wahe Guru Ji ka Khalsa, Wahe Guru Ji ki Fateh** means: "The Pure ones (*Khalsa*) belong to God (*Wahe Guru*), and all Victory (Fateh) belongs to God." *Ki* and *ka* are possessive pronouns. *Ji* means the soul (and is also a term of respect often added to the end of a person's name).

This whole mantra is a reminder to those who speak it and those who hear it, that we <u>all</u> belong to God, and God deserves the credit for any success (victory) we achieve. It affirms acknowledgment of God as the Doer and speaks to the aspiration of all yogis to surrender the little ego, in order to expand consciousness and awareness into the Universal. Remember, Khalsa are those who aspire to be pure in heart, clear in conscience, fearless, and effective in action, intuitive, kind, and compassionate, humble before the Infinite Creator, yet noble within the Self.

*Amritdhari* Sikhs (those who have taken the *Amrit* baptism, pledging to live as *Khalsa*) greet each other with this statement. Sikhs also shout it out quite frequently at certain times during the worship services in the *Gurdwara*, and sometimes spontaneously call it out to express enthusiasm and approval.

Ideally, *Wahe Guru Ji ka Khalsa, Wahe Guru Ji ki Fateh* keeps us humble.

# Bolay So Nihal

*Wahe Guru Ji ka Khalsa, Wahe Guru Ji ki Fateh* also follows another very frequently used call-and-answer expression of enthusiastic appreciation: *Bolay So Nihal*, which is answered by *Sat Siri Akaal*. *Bolay So Nihal* means, "All who answer this call will be blessed," while the *Sat Siri Akaal* response translates as, "Truth is great and undying." And who doesn't want to be blessed? So everyone shouts back *Sat Sri Akaal*! When people are super enthusiastic, this call and answer is repeated three to five times—after which **Wahe Guru Ji ka Khalsa, Wahe Guru Ji ki Fateh** follows.

# Drumming

Another sound you are likely to hear in some Gurdwaras is the rousing beat of a big kettledrum called a *Nagara*. This practice began several hundred years ago when Sikhs were often in encampments ready to go into battle. In 1684, Guru Gobind Singh Sahib got a special drum prepared. It was named "Ranjit" (the winner of the battlefield). This drum was beaten at Kesgarh Sahib Throne at Anandpur Sahib every day as a declaration of the sovereignty of the Sikh nation. Guru Gobind Singh made it obligatory that before the ending of Gurdwara, the *Nagara* must be beaten. *Nagara* is a symbol of sovereignty. Only the winner of a battle could beat it. *Nishan* (flag) and *Nagara* (drum) are an integral part of a *Takht* (Khalsa Throne), and you will see them at all Gurdwaras.

The *Nagara* is used in Gurdwaras for emphasis at certain points in the *Ardas* as the Gurdwara program is coming to a close. Remember, Sikhs are known as Warrior-Saints. (Read the story in the chapter about Guru Hargobind, the Sixth Nanak, to learn how and why Sikhs had to become warriors.)

# The Song of the Khalsa

### By MSS Livtar Singh Khalsa

*Ed. Note:*

*In 1975, Livtar Singh Khalsa (Atlanta, Georgia) composed this song recounting some of the major events in Sikh history. The Siri Singh Sahib directed that "The Song of the Khalsa" be sung in every Gurdwara immediately before the Anand Sahib. He even requested that the lyrics be inscribed on the back of his memorial marker. As a matter of historical interest, the words that were chiseled in stone were copied from an issue of "Beads of Truth," which unfortunately contained errors! Here are the actual words that Livtar wrote.*

1. Many speak of courage, speaking cannot give it.

    It's in the face of death that we must live it.

    When things are down and darkest

    That's when we stand tallest.

    Until the last star falls, we won't give an inch at all.


    (REFRAIN)

    Stand as the Khalsa: Strong as Steel, Steady as Stone

    Give our lives to God and Guru,

    Mind and soul, breath and bone


2. Guru Arjan gave his life to stand for what was right;

    He was burned and tortured five long days and nights.

    He could have stopped it anytime, just by giving in

    His strength a solid wall; he never gave an inch at all!

    Sons of the Khalsa, remember those who died,

    Stood their ground until their last breath

    So we who live now, might live free lives

*3. A princess is not royal by her birth or blood inside*

*But if her family's home is Anandpur Sahib,*

*She'll walk with such a grace and strength*

*The world will bow in awe*

*Until the mountains fall, she'll never give an inch at all!*

*Daughters of the Khalsa, in your strength our future lies,*

*Give our children fearless minds*

*To see the world through the Guru's eyes.*


*4. Baisakhi day we were thousands*

*But only five had the courage for dyin'.*

*Then one brave man, one flashing sword*

*Turned us all to lions.*

*And now we live his legacy to die before we fall,*

*And like the five who answered his call,*

*We can't turn back at all*

*(REFRAIN)*

5. The Tenth Guru gave even his sons

To give the Khalsa life.

His words stand like mountains

Against the winds of time:

That Khalsa will rule the world

All will be safe in its fold.

But if the Khalsa falls,
There won't be a world at all.


*(REFRAIN)*

Repeat "Sons of the Khalsa …

Repeat "Daughters of the Khalsa…

*(REFRAIN)*

Give our lives to God and Guru,

Mind and soul, are His alone.


*MSS Livtar Singh Khalsa (1975)*

# The Origins of Song of the Khalsa: A Recollection from the Artist

I have come full circle in understanding that "religion" gives you the lines on the side of the road to keep you headed in the right direction. Hopefully it also gives you the technology, the car to drive down that road. But once you arrive at the ONE, there are no Hindus, Muslims, and yes, Sikhs. There is only the One.

Now when I talk to people about it, they think I'm nuts. I talk in our local Indian Gurdwara and ask, "Was Guru Nanak a Sikh?" How could he be if there was no such "religion" at the time? Or my other favorite question for those being judgmental about who is a "good Sikh" or a "bad Sikh"—"On the day before Guru Nanak was born, how would one accomplish being a good Sikh?" You couldn't formally, but you could do all the things that have been the same since the beginning of time. Still, the question should never be, "Are you a good Sikh or bad Sikh or left Sikh or right Sikh?" The question is, "Are you doing those things that have liberated the beings since the beginning of time?" The Sikh path gives those rules and technology in the way they will be needed for the Aquarian Age, but it is our thing as humans to make them into cement instead of a flow.

There's a phrase I heard Sumpuran Singh (of Florida) use once. He said the founders of most religions usually don't start out to start a religion. They give a technique, a path; they attract a lot of students, and then later the followers "harden up" around the original concept. Once their minds have hardened up, then there are the usual walls… "They are on the other side, we are on this side. A is on that side, B is on this side." It defeats the whole original purpose, to get to One-ness.

I remember so clearly in our early days when we were so fanatical. The Siri Singh Sahib had to bring us through that experience to get clear of it. Since we are not in India, he gave us all our own version of how to "clean the floors of *Harimandir*." Somewhere in his teaching, for each person, there is that thing that is very hard to do (other than the usual yoga and sadhana, which are not easy). Yet if they do this thing, they will have their *karmas* cleaned and get the vision of third eye.

My version was to serve the sangat as ashram director, but more specifically, to serve the Gurdwara energy at our ashram in Atlanta. Because we weren't very large, everyone had to help for every Gurdwara. None of this once a month *missal* stuff for us. Plus every morning at sadhana there was a Gurdwara.

For the first ten years or so, I didn't like it, I just did it. Then I started to get the juice from it. I got more and more into it. This was my version of "cleaning the floors of the Golden Temple." This went on for years and years.

Then about three years ago, while I was driving my car, I suddenly knew I was One with the One. Not just intellectually, but in my total being. I saw the One everywhere in everything. I guess my third eye activated, though I'm not seeing *auras* or anything different than usual. All mental pain and self-doubt vanished in an instant, just like it says in the *Siri Guru Granth Sahib*. I saw the One doing every part in the play, and I knew that there isn't any part that isn't right. That includes me…I am absolutely perfect, and any thoughts that convey anything else are part of the illusion.

I no longer wondered if I was doing the right thing, or if I should be better at this, or worse at that. All of that self-nagging, which has no reality, was gone in an instant.

I was so shocked, I didn't know what to do. Why did it happen driving a car and not during some deep profound meditation?

In fact when it hit me in the car, I actually said, "Holy s**t, it really is all ONE!" (rather than something I would later have thought more appropriate). This concept of the One being and doing all…I had thought about it, meditated on it, read about it, and taught it. But when I actually saw it and merged into it…Wha!

After that I went almost mute for most of a year. There was no one to talk to, because there is no "other."

Finally, only because of the example of my teacher, I started talking again. He taught that there is no teacher, and no one to teach. He taught. Even though he said, "You think there is someone sitting here teaching, and you are sitting there listening. There is no such thing." He knew everything I knew, plus infinitely more, and still went through the game of life. So I literally copied his example to see where it would lead. I figure that's the next level.

I now hear his lectures totally differently. I understand what he is talking about (except for that "100,000 plus energy squared into the radiant angle of brain flexion" stuff), and I understand the role of dharma to get you there, but not to be your destination…just like he said so many times.

I became a "watcher," a word he used many times. I watch the movie now; I have no say.

It has slowed down my songwriting some, because the words would be something like, "One, One, One, One." I can't even use the point of view of me and Thou—that's not real. So I'll look to my teacher, I'll look to Guru Nanak and all the Gurus, and put my energy into sound and thought, so it can reflect back.

Maybe the most important thing I discovered was that the marble floors of Harimandir are all around us, not in a far away place. Just lean down, start scrubbing, and don't stop until you see the One in your reflection.

The "Song of the Khalsa" is from 1975. I always have to look it up by the movie that inspired it, "The Human Factor" starring George Kennedy.

That movie made me understand the term "fearless." Not overcoming fear, but being utterly without fear, the state of the enlightened.

I came home from the theatre, and I was so inspired I was almost agitated. I wanted to put it in some form that could be transmitted to others… to bottle it. That's how this song, through the filter of my sadhana and seva, came to be.

So leave the fear. Bani, Bana, Simran, and Seva can wash away any of that. Be in the flow and enjoy the "movie."

Long answer to a short question, but that title got me going.

Blessings and Love from Mr. and Mrs. Sonny[59]

---

[59]  Editor's Note: I've always called Livtar Singh by the affectionate nickname "Sonny" -SP

Livtar Singh sent me the rest of the story of the completion of the song itself:

I worked on the song in our sadhana room at the ashram. It took two or three hours, which is very quick for me. After I thought the song was finished, with four verses being written, I had a feeling of completion and great relief that it came out well. I decided to go upstairs to my bedroom and rest.

Just as I was passing through the doorway, I felt as if someone or something started knocking gently on my head, as you might knock lightly on a door.

Now this kind of thing may seem a little odd to you, but I was already familiar with many unusual experiences from my meditations. I took it right in stride and went along mentally.

"What?" (as in, "What do you want?"), I thought, somewhat defiantly. I could tell that since it had started out with head knocking, it was going to be some kind of bugging, not hugging.

"You're not finished with the song," 'It' said.

"What do you mean? It's good, it says what I felt, and it has **four whole verses**. That's plenty!" I thought back emphatically.

Surely the blazing logic of my argument that, "It's the number of verses that counts," would overcome any further objection. It was happening so suddenly I wasn't quite realizing yet that whoever could communicate with me internally probably already knew how many verses there were.

"No, it's not done!" 'It' insisted in my head.

There is a kind of a birthing process involved for me to write a song, and this 'It' was telling me it wasn't good enough.

Even so, it finally got through to me that this exchange was something new and different. Am I hearing from one of the Gurus? Siri Singh Sahib? My own soul? God? What? The one thing I knew was that it was not my own mind. I was having an actual "conversation" with someone else.

"Are you sure?" I gave one more hopeful try.

"Go finish it," 'It' vibrated in me.

I realized that I should listen and not argue.

"Oh, all right, have it your way," I thought (still a little peevishly).

I went back downstairs and picked up my guitar. Immediately, out popped one more verse, easy as bowing your head. The verse was "Baisakhi day we were thousands." I rearranged the song a little, and that new verse then became the fourth verse.

I went back upstairs. I stopped in front of the door and waited a moment. Then I passed through expectantly, my eyes looking up to either side of me.

There were no more head bops. There was no more communication from 'It.' 'It' was satisfied, and so was I.

To this day I have no idea who or what 'It' was. Nothing like that has ever happened again. I just accept it and give thanks for that clear command, and give thanks that I could hear.

P.S. Intuitively, I have always "suspected" it was Siri Singh Sahib Ji. He never confirmed or denied.

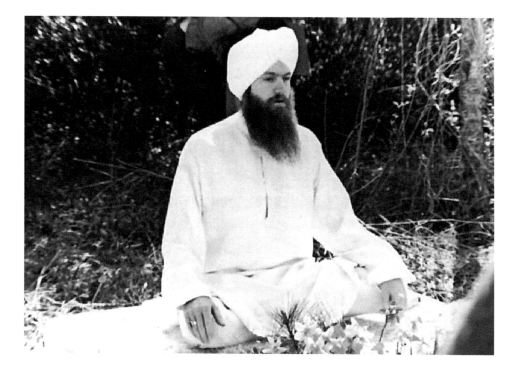

*MSS Livtar Singh Khalsa (1976)*

# Anand Sahib – The Song of Bliss

After the *Song of the Khalsa* and before the Ardas it is customary in every Gurdwara to sing *Anand Sahib*, the joyful "Song of Bliss" composed by Guru Amar Das, the Third Guru.

Here are some excerpts from a talk about the *Anand Sahib* by the Siri Singh Sahib.

. . . . . . . . . . . . . . . . . . . . . . . . . . . . . . . . . . . . . . . . . . . . . . . . . . . . . . . . . . . . . . . . . . . . . . .

*"There are a lot of literary meanings of the stage of Anand. In English, you have an equivalent of it called "bliss." Anand can be attached to any state where you momentarily feel satisfied. That's why Guru Amar Das wrote Anand Sahib — the command, the domain of the Anand.*

*"The Anand of which Guru Amar Das speaks is described in the Bible as "the peace which passeth all understanding." So it really is not simply a joyful state, but a state of profound spiritual bliss which is all-pervasive and beyond the power of words to describe. Therein lies the "Catch 22." Unless you have actually experienced it, you can't understand what he is talking about. Anand Sahib is Guru Amar Das' expression of the unspeakable joy of that state of Being. In it he is truly telling that story, which can never be told.*

*"Therefore, please read Anand Sahib as an instruction. Understand its capacity and depth. It's very educational. The easiest and most educational Bani, which a person can read and understand, is the Anand Sahib.*

*"Follow its words. Ask yourself questions. Befriend it. Practice it and live it. You will not have to find anything else. You will realize what you have, and what Guru Amar Das gave you as the best gift.*

*"It's my prayer and my feeling that we who follow the path of the Shabd shall speak words which we honor. We who follow the word of the Shabd will honor what we do, and we who are the Sikhs shall honor our being, our existence, and our Inner Self, so that the world around us can totally understand who we are.*

*"Sikh Dharma is based on one fundamental thing. That at the cost of your life, at the cost of your comfort, even at the cost of you, you must understand that whatever you speak must be worthy of trust, even by the standard of your worst arch-enemy. That is what a Sikh is about.*

*"Therefore, please understand, Anand is not in having too much money. Neither is it in too much power. Neither is it in too much beauty and neither is it in too much destruction.*

*"There's no joy except seeing your own soul within your own self with your Inner Eye. What I am saying is not difficult."*

. . . . . . . . . . . . . . . . . . . . . . . . . . . . . . . . . . . . . . . . . . . . . . . . . . . . . . . . . . . . . . . . . . . . . . .

**Ed. Note:**
*The Anand Sahib is included in the Siri Guru Granth Sahib. In it, the Guru is talking to his Mind, telling it what to do. Guru Amar Das calls himself "Nanak," for he is speaking from the same level of divine consciousness as the First Guru.*

. . . . . . . . . . . . . . . . . . . . . . . . . . . . . . . . . . . . . . . . . . . . . . . . . . . . . . . . . . . . . . . . . . . . . . .

# EXCERPTS FROM THE *ANAND SAHIB*

## *Translated by SS Ek Ong Kaar Kaur Khalsa*

Mind of mine—
Always be with the Essence of the Divine
Inside your own heart
And inside of everything
Around you.

Be with
The Essence of the Divine
Inside yourself
And inside all things,
My mind.

This will cause you to forget
All your pains and sorrows.

Feel the Divine Essence
Present
In every fiber of your being.

Feel yourself
As one fiber
In the vast weave of life.

Intermingle
And surrender your identity
To and with the Divine.

Then,
The Creator will do
All of your work

*For you*
*And bring all your affairs*
*To completion.*

*That powerful Master*
*Is in control*
*Of all the things*
*That concern and worry you.*

*So why ever*
*Let yourself*
*Forget that One?*

*Says Nanak—*
*Mind of mine—*
*Always be with the Essence of the Divine*
*Inside your own heart*
*And inside of everything*
*Around you.*

*Says Nanak,*
*Listen you who live*
*By your purity,*
*Spiritual discipline*
*And grace*

*Keep it with you, Beloved Ones.*
*The Sound Current*
*That cuts*
*The ego-shackles of the mind.*

*Trusting and following*
*The command*
*Of the Teacher*

> Sing in the
> Frequency and vibration
> Which will bring you the experience
> Of Ultimate Reality

*Ed. Note:*
*The complete Anand Sahib has a total of forty verses.*

# ARDAS: *The Power Of Prayer*

The Siri Singh Sahib used to say that the only real power a human has is the power of his or her prayer. What is prayer? It is when the finite being speaks to the Infinite from the heart and soul, asking for help, guidance, or healing. And the Infinite listens.

Meditation is where the Infinite can speak to the finite through the sixth *chakra*, or center of consciousness—the intuition, and the finite listens deeply. There is a two-way communication. When we chant and pray in a group, with a focused collective consciousness, we get that exponential effect which makes our prayer that much more powerful.

Yogi Bhajan also often said, "In order to reach Universal Consciousness, you have to go from individual consciousness through group consciousness."

A friend of Yogi Bhajan's who visited Guru Ram Das Ashram told us about some of his harrowing mountain climbing experiences. He said that he always started each climb by reciting the traditional Sikh prayer, *Ardas*—including a personal prayer for protection. In all his years of rough terrain and extremely hazardous expeditions, he had never had an accident.[60]

The *Ardas* is a vital part of every Sikh's life. It is a perfect formula of prayer of the heart, and can be done any time, anywhere, whether at home, at a board meeting, or in the Gurdwara—where it is always recited just before the *Hukam* is taken.

*Ardas* is always done out loud, and Sikhs always offer an *Ardas* to begin any major event, and even some minor ones. The *Ardas* has a standard format, including, but not limited to, remembering the Sikh Gurus and recalling the courage of all those who sacrificed to preserve this path. It always ends with a phrase that wishes good and blessings to *everyone* in the world.

---

[60] Ed. Note – The middle part of the translated Ardas that appears here refelects common addtions that have been made by
Sikhs during the 19th and 20th centuries. This portion is optional and is indented.
Book: *Miracles of Ardaas — Incredible Adventures and Survivals*, by M. S. Kohli, 2003

Though the beginning (up through the mention of Guru Tegh Bahadur) and ending of the *Ardas* (…O Nanak, those who know their True Identity ever live in ecstasy and excellence…) were given by Guru Gobind Singh, space is provided in the middle for the spoken and unspoken prayers of everyone gathered to flow through the *ardasee,* the one whose voice is speaking the prayer aloud. The prayer is the collective prayer of everyone gathered together at that moment in time and space. In this way, specific blessings such as healing and protection can be invoked. Usually there is a piece of paper on which people can write their requests for special prayers for healing, or birthday blessings, or on the occasion of a death—in which latter case the everyone chants *"AKAAL"* several times to speed the departed soul on its way to God.

Anyone can offer the *Ardas*, either in English (or the local language) or in the original *Gurmukhi*.

## An English Translation of the Ardas: Sikh Prayer

*Remember the Primal Power. Think of Guru Nanak, then of Guru Angad and Amar Das and Ram Das! Remember Arjan, Hargobind and holy Har Rai. Think of the blessed Harkrishan, whose sight dispels all sorrows. Remember Tegh Bahadur, and the nine treasures shall run to our homes. There are all with us everywhere. May the Tenth King, Guru Gobind Singh, protect us everywhere.*

*Blessed, blessed, O Khalsa Ji, is the Guru Granth Sahib, the Light of all. With the light of the Guru in your heart, call on God!*

*Wahe Guru!*

*The Five Beloved Ones, the four sons of the Tenth Master, the Forty Liberated Ones, and all those who kept up in the face of tyranny and oppression: think of their deeds O Khalsa Ji and call on God!*

*Wahe Guru!*

*All those men and women who, keeping the Name in their hearts, rose in the amrit vela to remember and merge with the One; who shared their earnings with others; who defended those who could not defend themselves; who stood fast through all the tests of time and space; who saw others' faults but looking only to their souls served them anyway; think of their deeds, O Khalsa Ji and call on God!*

*Wahe Guru!*

*Those who allowed themselves to be cut up limb by limb, who had their scalps scraped off, who were broken on the wheel, who were sawn in half or flayed alive, but who never gave up their faith and never betrayed their own soul, but remained steadfast till their last breath, think of their sweet resignation, O Khalsa Ji and call on God!*

*Wahe Guru!*

*Meditate on the Gurudwaras, the thrones of religious authority, and all the places blessed by the touch of the Gurus' feet. O Khalsa Ji, call on God!*

**Wahe Guru!**

*Now let the whole Khalsa offer our prayer together.*

*Let the whole Khalsa remember the Naam.*

*As we think of Him, may we feel completely blessed.*

*Wahe Guru!*

*Wahe Guru!*

*Wahe Guru!*

*May God's protection and grace extend to all the bodies of the Khalsa, wherever we may be.*

*May the Lord's glory be fulfilled and His will prevail.*

*May all our homes and endeavors be blessed with success.*

*May the sword of God assist us.*

*May the Khalsa always triumph.*

*May our Sangats, flags, and Gurdwaras abide forever and ever,*

*May the kingdom of justice prevail.*

*May we be blessed with the sight of the Holy Harimandir Sahib and the sip and dip of its holy pool of Nectar.*

*May all Sikhs be united in love.*

*May the hearts of the Sikhs be humble, but their wisdom be exalted in the keeping of the Lord, O Khalsa Ji, say that God is Great!*

*Wahe Guru!*

*O true King, O beloved Father, we have sung the sweet hymns, we heard Thy life-giving Word and have meditated on Thy manifold blessings. May these things find a loving place in our hearts and serve to draw our souls closer and closer towards Thee. May all the silent prayers of our hearts be fulfilled by Thy grace.*

*Save us from lust, wrath, greed, pride and attachment; and keep us always and only attached to Thy Lotus Feet.*

*Grant to all Thy Sikhs the gift of Sikh Dharma, the gift of long hair, the gift of faith and confidence in Thee, the gift of reading and understanding Thy Gurbani, and most of all, the gift of Thy Holy Name*

*O kind Father; O loving Father, By Thy grace we have spent the night in peace and happiness; and risen to meditate on Thee and listen to Thy Holy Word. Grant that we may always do what is right according to Thy Will.*

*Grant us light and understanding so that we may know what pleases Thee. We offer this prayer in Thy presence O wonderful Lord:*

*Forgive our mistakes and help us to keep ourselves pure.*

*Let us be in the company of only people of love, so we may always remember Thy Name.*

*O Nanak, those who know their True Identity ever live in ecstasy and excellence. Through the Power of Thy Bani, may the whole world be blessed to live in this way.*

*Wahe Guru Ji ka Khalsa, Wahe Guru Ji ki Fateh!*

Chapter Nine

# Commitment and Fulfillment

☬

## KHALSA CONSCIOUSNESS AND THE FIVE K'S

When people realize they want to live their lives in accordance with definite principles that match those of Sikh Dharma, they often decide to make a spiritual commitment by taking vows. Taking vows is like getting lifetime insurance against compromising one's principles for convenience. Sikh Dharma has two levels of commitment: Sikh Vows and *Amrit Sanchar*.

# Sikh Vows

Sikh Vows are simple statements of commitment to self-discipline and surrender to the *Shabd Guru* as our highest Guide to spiritual awakening.

Sikh Vows provide a foundation of living a certain lifestyle to further develop and enhance our spiritual practice. The vows include not cutting our hair; refraining from meat, alcohol, and other stimulants; remaining celibate until married and maintaining a monogamous relationship with our spouse; and committing to meditation and prayer each day.

# The Amrit Sanchar: Becoming Khalsa

The most powerful vows on the path of Sikh Dharma are taken in the *Amrit Sanchar* (ceremony). The word *amrit* is often translated into English as "nectar," but the root sounds of the word literally mean, "Deathless Blood." Therefore, receiving *Amrit* grants a state of consciousness where a person knows in the very marrow of their bones that the physical body and the mind are temporary—so that they are beyond the power of death; and that the eternal, undying Spirit within each one of us is *who we truly are.*

Sikhs who have taken these vows are called *Amrit Dhari* and take the last name of *Khalsa*, meaning "pure one."

Let's go back to 1699, at the *Baisakhi* celebration where the first *Amrit* was given by Guru Gobind Singh, the Tenth Sikh Guru.

# The Birth of the Khalsa

Baisakhi was already celebrated as a joyous springtime (April-May) renewal of life celebration when, over 300 years ago, in 1699, Guru Gobind Singh sent messages to all the local Sikh communities that everyone should come in large numbers at Anandpur Sahib to celebrate Baisakhi together. He stood before the assembly of about 80,000 people with an unsheathed sword and his voice rang out, "I need a head. Who will offer me their head?" This was high drama, asking his Sikhs to make the supreme sacrifice. He repeated his shocking challenge five times in all.

Hearing this, most of the people in the crowd got scared and ran away, but one at a time, five brave and devoted Sikhs came forward. One at a time they disappeared into the Master's tent with him (and his sword), finally to emerge unscathed. Thereupon the Guru called them his Panj Piaray, his "Five Beloved Ones." The Guru stirred an iron bowl full of water with a double-edged sword called a khanda, while chanting over the water to fill it with sacred vibrations. As the water was being stirred, Mata Sahib Kaur, the Guru's wife, added Patashas (sugar crystals) to the bowl. The Guru then gave this sweet ambrosia to the five Sikhs who had volunteered their heads. He gave them the name "Singh," meaning "lion," to be followed with "Khalsa."

Later, the Guru himself knelt before the five and asked them to give the Amrit to him. Thus the Guru became the disciple of his Sikhs—and Guru Gobind Rai became Guru Gobind Singh. He baptized Sikhs to be pure and explained the way of life of purity, and then he said, *"Rehit piaaraa moeh ko, Sikh piaaraa naa-eh."* Rehit, this way of life, the dharma, the call of duty, is precious to me... not any Sikh. He didn't reject the Sikhs. He just improved them. He gave them a simple, pure lifestyle, and the rights and blessings that come with it.

Now Sikhs all over the world gather on or about April 14th every year to celebrate this historic birthday of the Khalsa.

## Description of the Amrit Ceremony

The *Amrit Sanchar* re-creates the experience from the first Baisakhi. You might call it the baptism of Khalsa. Those who receive *Amrit* commit to becoming protectors and custodians of the Universal Truths held within the *Siri Guru Granth Sahib* and, in fact, protectors of those who cannot protect themselves. They also embody the spiritual way of life that the Sikh Masters created. Those who receive Amrit commit to surrender everything – body, mind, property, and life – to preserve these values and this eternal wisdom.

The ceremony takes place during the *Amrit Vela*—the hours before sunrise. Five people who have already received *Amrit* serve to represent the original *Panj Piaray*, the five Beloved Ones.

Gathering together in the *Gurdwara*, the candidates for receiving Amrit meditate while the *Panj Piaray* each recite one of the five *Banis* (daily Sikh prayers) while stirring water and sugar in an iron bowl with a *khanda (double-edged sword.)* The power of the sacred vibrations infuses the water and alters its molecular structure. The frequency of the *Shabd* enters the water and transforms it into *Amrit* [61] A few drops of *Amrit* are sprinkled on the top of the heads of each candidate five times while they repeat *Wahe Guru Ji ka Khalsa, Wahe Guru Ji ki Fateh*[62]. Thus committing to live as Khalsa, those receiving the Amrit are then given the nectar to drink. This commitment offered in the Amrit Sanchar ceremony opens the door for a person to be able to manifest inherent purity and light in every aspect of life. This is the inner experience of *Khalsa*.

# The Amrit Vows

Those taking *Amrit* are instructed as follows:

- The *Mul Mantra*[63] is your Root Mantra. It gives you your foundation, and serves as an anchor in your life.

- The Guru Mantra is *Wahe Guru*. It expresses your state of ecstasy and helps you to fulfill your destiny.

- You have taken rebirth in the family of the *Khalsa*, and therefore your spiritual father is Guru Gobind Singh, your spiritual mother is Mata Sahib Kaur, and your birthplace is Anandpur Sahib.

- Men take the surname of *Singh* (Lion). Your new identity is fearlessness.

- Women take the surname of *Kaur* (Princess or Lioness). Your new identity is one of grace and fearlessness. Both men and women take the family name of *Khalsa*. You have joined the family of the Pure Ones.

At the first *Amrit* ceremony, Guru Gobind Singh gave the *Rehit*, or self-discipline, which was recorded and passed down through the generations. This includes wearing five symbols, called the Five K's.

# The Five K's

When the father of the *Khalsa*, Guru Gobind Singh, gave the gift of the five K's, he did so with a promise. He promised that if we follow his teachings and keep ourselves distinct, we will have his power and support. Here is a description of the significance of each of the five K's.

## Kara – Steel Bracelet

*Kara* is a steel or iron bracelet that women wear on the left wrist and men wear on the right wrist. The *kara* symbolizes that we are never a slave to any man. We bow only to God, and serve only Infinity. The *kara* is a reminder to keep the power of steel in our *aura*. The steel reminds us that when our strength is tested, our commitment shall never falter. The *kara* is round, symbolizing our oneness with the Infinite, the boundless, undying, Almighty God, the *Akal Purkh*.

[61] *Messages from Water* by Masaru Emoto (Vol. 2) (scientific experiments verify the effect of sounds on/in water).
[62] "The Pure Ones (Khalsa) belong to God: all victory belongs to God."
[63] Mool Mantra: see page 56.

# Kesh – Uncut Hair

We do not cut our hair. It is God's gift, giving us sensitivity, power, and protection, so we keep our hair in its natural form. We protect our hair by coiling it in a Rishi knot on the crown center at the top of the head and we cover our heads with a turban when we are in public.

Each person's hair grows to a particular length—which is the correct length for that person. It takes approximately three years after the last time hair has been cut for antennae to form at the tips of the hair. These antennae serve to draw in greater quantities of vitamin D from the sun as well as other more subtle forms of cosmic energy.

Yogi Bhajan taught that if a person, from birth to the end, does not ruin the antenna, *the hair,* then insanity cannot come near that person under any circumstance.

When the hair of humans was cut for the first time, it was considered a punishment. In the tribal wars, when one tribe conquered the other tribe, the seriously wounded were killed. Those who were healthy were made slaves. They would cut the women's hair and shave the men's heads as the sign of slavery. That was considered so totally unfortunate that some women committed suicide rather than subject themselves to getting their hair cut. The full length of the hair on the head and keeping all the locks intact constituted dignity and freedom.

When you cut your hair, you deprive yourself of your rightful God-given strength and vitality. The prophets in the Old Testament knew this when they retold the story of Samson. Native Americans have always known it. Little children may intuitively know this when, kicking and screaming, they are forced by their parents to sit in the barber's chair for their first haircut. Somehow the "flower children of the sixties," as they were called, also knew it. Many of them today have become *Khalsa,* but they had already decided not to cut their hair, before they heard the Guru's message.

# Kanga – Wooden Comb

We keep a wooden comb in our hair under the turban as part of our commitment to keep our physical world and ourselves graceful and clean. We balance our electromagnetic energy when we comb our hair with a wooden comb. Combing the hair with a wooden comb up, back, forward, and so on, encourages strong circulation and stimulation of the scalp and enhances health, energy, and longevity.

# Kirpan – Sacred Sword

We also wear the *kirpan,* a small sacred sword. Literally meaning "kindness," the *kirpan* is to be used only in self-defense or to protect those who are unable to defend themselves.

. . . . . . . . . . . . . . . . . . . . . . . . . . . . . . . . . . . . . . . . . . . . . . . . . . . . . .

*"Guru Gobind Singh made it binding for Khalsa to wear a Kirpan. It is a symbol, and symbolically you must wear a kirpan. The sword is the symbol for all arms, and it is the symbol of our reverence for the sacredness of*

*all weapons. If you are made to worship arms, then you also know how to respect arms. You will never misuse them. When you worship the sword, then you will be subconsciously the last person to use the sword. You will be the most restrictive. You cannot madly play with something that is sacred. Have you ever seen any man in his madness throw his altar out of the window? Never. When a person can do that, he is not human."*

*-Yogi Bhajan*

Guru Gobind Singh promised us when we keep our Khalsa form, wear a *kirpan* and hold it sacred, we would always be protected as if there were 125,000 soldiers at our side. We can never be harmed by that which we hold as sacred.

## Kachhera – Special cotton underwear (under-shorts)

Under shorts are worn as protection and a reminder to keep the creative sexual energy in balance. We honor the sacredness of our sexual energy and all our relationships. We only have sexual relations with our spouse, and we relate to all other men and women either as our sons, daughters, brothers, sisters, mothers, or fathers.

*"The under shorts were purposefully designed to create a protective air pocket around the genitals and the hips. The hip joint is the largest area in the entire body where the bones contact a rich bed of capillaries. This is where the calcium balance of the body is maintained. When this area is protected, and a constant temperature is kept, the calcium regulation is correct. The first four vertebrae are contained in that air pocket. In this protection, one enjoys the creative energy in life." -*

*- Yogi Bhajan*

# THE PATH OF THE SOLDIER SAINT

## *What is a Soldier-Saint?*
## *It is a Spiritual Warrior*

Sikhs are encouraged to learn and practice martial arts to help them conquer their fear and become non-violent in the truest sense of the word: without fear and without anger *(nirbhao, nirvair)*. The principle of true *ahimsa* (non-violence) is to actively prevent violence, not to simply stand by idly while violence is being done. To that end, a Sikh assumes the responsibility for preventing violence and for protecting a defenseless person. That is done with the minimum force required. Most often, words can resolve the problem because of a Sikh's forceful projection. If a Sikh is forced to fight, it is always in self-defense or defense of another person, never in aggression.

The spiritual practice of martial arts originated in the Orient and has more recently spread to the West. A fundamental tenet of martial arts training is that a martial artist never initiates violence, but redirects violent energy directed against him in order to neutralize a destructive attack.

In the time of Guru Gobind Singh, Sikhs were under frequent attack by chieftains and emperors who were only interested in earthly power and material gain. The Guru's army was often victorious in the face of almost incredible odds, and was always kind and compassionate to wounded enemies, and to the families of enemies killed in battle. Guru Gobind Singh himself dealt with his opponents with grace, compassion, wisdom, and strength. To the spiritual warrior, the true enemies are fear, ignorance, hatred, and the illusion of separateness. The symbol of the sword (kirpan) reminds us to cut through this illusion with courage, clarity, and strength.

# Another Way to Serve

. . . . . . . . . . . . . . . . . . . . . . . . . . . . . . . . . . . . . . . . . . . . . . . . . . . . . . . . . . . . .

## Excerpts from
## What Is the Sikh Dharma Ministry Today?

*By SS Dr. Sat-Kaur Khalsa,*
*Secretary of Religion for Sikh Dharma*

Back in the 1970s, as the Siri Singh Sahib, Yogi Bhajan established a Sikh Ministry in the West—another level of commitment for those who are called to serve as Ministers.

He explained the structure emphasizing that it is not a hierarchy. In fact, he told us, "Visualize an inverted pyramid."

On the very bottom, the lowest position, supporting the entire structure was the Siri Singh Sahib (and he surely served us all!). The next tier is composed of those who have Administrative duties; they are titled Mukhia Singh Sahibs and Mukhia Sardarni Sahibas (MSS). Their job is to support the Singh Sahibs and Sardarni Sahibas (male and female ministers, SS) above them, whose responsibility is to serve the Sadh Sangat directly. Finally, he said that the most important people in the pyramid are the ones on the top level. They are the people we are to serve. They have no titles, and they may not even be Sikhs. This structure establishes that, as ministers, we are here to serve all of humanity.

. . . . . . . . . . . . . . . . . . . . . . . . . . . . . . . . . . . . . . . . . . . . . . . . . . . . . . . . . . . . .

We are servants of the spiritual family of Sikhs worldwide.

The relationship between a Sikh and his Guru is direct, no person stands in between, least of all us (ministers).

We do not financially benefit in any way from Dasvandh (tithing) or the donations given in the Gurdwara.

All people are equal before God, and the titles (Singh Sahib, Sardarni Sahiba, etc.) give us no special position or privileges.

To be a minister means we are the first to step forward, the first to offer whatever is needed, the last to eat, the last to sleep.

. . . . . . . . . . . . . . . . . . . . . . . . . . . . . . . . . . . . . . . . . . . . . . . . . . . . . . . . . . . . .

Today, the Ministry is a vibrant, richly diversified body of leaders. In addition to performing weddings, last rites, and counseling, each Minister brings his or her God-given gifts to serve the needs of our communities. It is as if every Minister is a unique "patch," all of which, when sewn together with the Guru's Word, produce a quilt that covers the needs of the world. *Seva*—selfless service—is the theme and code by which Sikh Dharma Ministers aspire to live.

Sikh Dharma Ministers serve as chaplains in hospitals, healing centers, universities, and airports. They are active in the United Nations and interfaith organizations, such as the World Parliament of Religions. Ministers may be found in many service areas in inner cities, shelters, and, of course, in Gurdwaras. Sikh Ministers teach, feed people, help with substance abuse recovery, and uplift people in a variety of ways.

To find a local Sikh Dharma Minister, please contact SS Ek Ong Kar Kaur Khalsa in the Chancellor's Office, Los Angeles, CA: ekongkarkaurkhalsa@earthlink.net

Chapter Ten

# A Householder Path

☬

## Spiritual Community: Sadh Sangat

One of the most important supports for someone who embarks on a spiritual path is a community of people practicing the same set of teachings, living and working together with the same values and consciousness. This is called the Sadh Sangat, literally the "community of the disciplined ones."

From the beginning, Yogi Bhajan always said that he had not come here to gather students, but to create teachers. In the early 1970s, as more and more of us came to study with him, he began to send people to various cities in North America and Europe to set up ashrams and begin to teach Kundalini Yoga and share the teachings of the Guru.

An ashram is a place where people come to live together to study and practice a spiritual path. At first, most of us were young and unmarried, and often an ashram would take the form of one large house with many rooms, single women sharing a space together separate from the single men. The largest room would become the room where we practiced our morning sadhana, or daily spiritual practice, and it often did double duty as our Gurdwara as we began to learn more of the teachings of Sikh Dharma. Food was purchased, cooked, and eaten communally, and all chores were organized and shared as "karma yoga," the yoga of action.

As time went by, we began to get married and start families. At that point the "one big house" model didn't work so well and we developed communities where many families lived near each other and shared space for morning sadhana, Gurdwara, and community gatherings. In some cities we were able to start family (3HO Family) businesses and yoga centers, which could offer employment to ashram members and also provide a way for us to interact with the larger community. An ashram community is a place for people to come who want to learn about and experience this path and these teachings.

*Saadh Sangat* means a gathering of people who do sadhana! *Saadhaks*. Living in a spiritual community is the conscious choice to be with people who elevate you, inspire you, and support your own sadhana and spiritual lifestyle. It is about choosing "who you hang with." Do you choose to "have a few beers with the guys" and try to blend in and be like everyone else, or do you choose to spend time with others who are also working on themselves and living a conscious, spiritual lifestyle? There's an old saying, "You're only as good as the company you keep." Or, how about, "Birds of a feather flock together."

# Women and Sikh Dharma

Long before Women's Lib, long before women gained the right to vote in the Western world, over 500 years ago, Guru Nanak spoke of the importance and value of women. His famous words on the subject are recorded in the *Siri Guru Granth Sahib:*

*We are born of a woman, we are conceived in the womb of a woman, we are engaged and married to a woman. We make friends with women, and the generations continue because of women. When one woman dies, we take another one. We are bound with the world through women. Why should we talk ill of she who gives birth to kings? Everyone is born from a woman. No one exists without her. Only the eternal formless One is beyond gender.*

Guru Nanak Dev, Var Asa, p. 473

The traditional Sikh prayer, the *Ardas,* recited by Sikhs all over the world, begins with this invocation: "After first worshipping the *Adi Shakti* (the 'Primal power')...." *Shakti* is God's power in manifestation. It is the feminine, creative aspect of God. Every woman is a goddess, a "Shakti."

Sikh history is rich with stories of courageous and noble women. When forty of Guru Gobind Singh's soldiers decided that they didn't want to fight anymore, and literally ran home to their wives, their women sent them back into battle. The fighting to overcome the Mughal invaders on December 29, 1705 had been hard and desperate. In spite of their overwhelming numbers, the Mughal troops failed to capture Guru Gobind Singh and had to retire in defeat. The major part in this battle was played by this group of forty Sikhs who had deserted the Guru at Anandpur during the long siege, but who, scolded by their wives at home, had come back to redeem themselves under the leadership of a brave and devoted woman, Mai Bhago. Fighting desperately to stop the enemy's advance toward the Guru's position, they fell. The Guru blessed them, calling them the "Forty Liberated Ones." The site is now marked by a sacred shrine and a pool of water infused with the sound current of *Gurbani.* The town which has grown around them is called Muktsar, the "Pool of Liberation."

Guru Gobind Singh had a great reverence for the feminine creative power *(Adi Shakti)*. When he created the *Khalsa* in 1699, he said that *Khalsa* "has no gender." He asked his wife, Mata Sahib Kaur, to prepare the amrit (sweet nectar) to balance the strength of the steel used in the ceremony. Over the years, political, cultural, and social influences have affected the practices of the Sikh path in India, and women are denied participating in all areas of service to the Sikh Panth. In particular, a lot of politics surrounds the upkeep of the Gurdwaras. Considering that one of our most basic beliefs is equality of gender, it's really sad to see the "old guard" still excluding women from the privilege of washing the floors of the Golden Temple every night.

A heartfelt poem and painting by SS Gurukirin Kaur Khalsa relates the longing of women to do seva inside the Golden Temple.

# Pure Longing

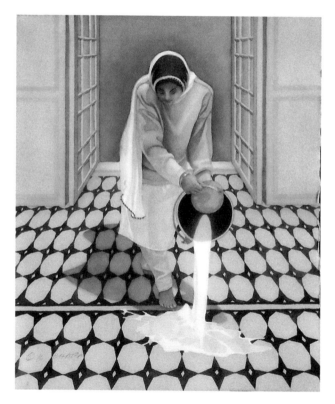

*Harimandir Sahib longs for the touch of Thy mothers,*

*Thy sisters, daughters, and all the others,*

*Who bow each day to Siri Guru Granth,*

*Following the path of the Khalsa Panth,*

*Who enter freely through all four doors,*

*Except when it is time to clean the floors.*

*In those holiest hours when it is such*

*A beautiful time to serve and touch*

*The marble where the saints have walked,*

*Why must those gilded doors be locked*

*To women alone, the Guru's daughters,*

*Cleansed by Thy Word and Thy Holy Waters?*

*The women of Bibi Bhani's line,*

*And those descended from Mata Sahib Kaur's time,*

*Gather as one to utter this prayer:*

*"O compassionate Guru of infinite care,*

*Let all Sikhs enact this holy rite,*

*As all are immaculate in Thy sight."*

# What Yogi Bhajan Taught About Women

When Yogi Bhajan came to the West, he did not bring with him any social or cultural bias excluding women from any aspect of Sikh Dharma. Here, both men and women are ministers and *granthis*. Both men and women can and do perform any and all types of service for their Guru and the congregation. As a Teacher, Yogi Bhajan devoted a great deal of his time and energy to awaken women from all spiritual paths to their own dignity, divinity, grace, and power. He reminded us often that the future of the planet depends upon the consciousness of women! One of his favorite sayings was, "When a man falls, an individual falls. When a woman falls, a generation falls." He taught that the consciousness and vibration of a mother is the most powerful influence on her child, especially while it is in the womb and during the first three years of life.

*"The highest incarnation of God is the female, through which God can take birth. All the avatars, all sages, all messengers of God, all messiahs never dropped directly from the sky. It is one womb of one woman which can give you the Godhead. There is a very popular saying in the scriptures: The strength of God is unlimited and is that of a woman."*

*-Yogi Bhajan, June 30, 1983*

# *Marriage*

The Sikh way of life is the life of a householder—creating cozy homes filled with warmth, family, and children.

Married life is both a powerful tool for personal and spiritual growth, as well as a deep source of satisfaction. The household is the backbone of a stable society. It is known as the *Ghrist Ashram*, the highest state of living, in which husband and wife live as one soul in two bodies. *Karmas* are shared, and each spouse mirrors the other and supports the other. It is a most mutual situation. Have you ever looked up the word "marry" in the dictionary? One of the definitions is "to combine suitably or agreeably; to blend flavors together" as in, "marry the milk and honey together." When milk and honey are "married" they cannot be separated, for the two separate things have become a different, third thing that combines the qualities of both.

## *Sikh Weddings: A Ceremony of Commitment*

Sikh weddings are really beautiful, and can run the gamut from extremely formal, to being intimate and cozy, with the sangat (congregation) actively participating, and the minister questioning the couple very personally regarding their sincerity and commitment before the "official" ceremony begins.

After the couple has been questioned by the Minister, and everyone is satisfied that the wedding should proceed, there is a traditional *shabd* (sacred verse) played and sung by the musicians, and the bride and groom stand up and prepare to walk together holding a *palay* (shawl), with the man leading, as they circle clockwise around the *Siri Guru Granth Sahib* before returning to their places in front of the Guru, where they bow in acknowledgement of their acceptance of the instructions stated in that verse. The couple makes four such rounds, circumnavigating the Guru—symbolic of the fact that the Guru is the center, the pivotal guidance for their married life. Each round refers to a stage of marriage. The first round is about leaving the past behind and starting a new spiritual life together. The second round is about making the Guru the center of your marriage. The third round is about serving the *Sadh Sangat* (spiritual community) and relying on their support. The final round says that marriage is a carriage to carry you to your destination of liberation and merger with the One. After each round, the couple bows together to the Guru, pledging to use these principles as the foundation for their married life. It's a very definite lifetime commitment to base their relationship on love of God and Guru.

Many years ago, SS Shanti Kaur Khalsa questioned the Siri Singh Sahib, Yogi Bhajan, about the practice of having the man leading the woman, with the shawl wrapped over the man's shoulder, and the woman holding it from behind him. She thought this was some old non-Sikh practice and was wondering why we do this, making the woman seem subservient by *following* the man.

The first answer that Yogi Bhajan gave Shanti, with a chuckle, was, "Well, someone has to go first." Of course, she wasn't satisfied with that answer. When she persisted, he replied, "It is all in your point of view.

You see the woman following the man subserviently. What I see is that marriage is a carriage in which the husband and wife ride to Infinity together. The horse is in front, and the driver sits behind and holds the reins."

He was teaching her that there are many levels of meaning. Interpretation depends upon our preconceived ideas and personal perspective. People filter things through their own frame of reference.

. . . . . . . . . . . . . . . . . . . . . . . . . . . . . . . . . . . . . . . . . . . . . . . . . . . . . . . . . . . . . . . . . . . . . . . . . .

For his own wedding, Guru Ram Das wrote a wedding song in four verses called the *Lavan*. It is found on page 773 of the *Siri Guru Granth Sahib*.

. . . . . . . . . . . . . . . . . . . . . . . . . . . . . . . . . . . . . . . . . . . . . . . . . . . . . . . . . . . . . . . . . . . . . . . . . .

# THE WEDDING CEREMONY:
## *LAVAN* – ENGLISH TRANSLATION

*1. In the first round of the marriage ceremony, the Lord gives you His Instructions for performing the daily duties of married life. Instead of performing rituals by routine, embrace the righteous life of Dharma, and do nothing that separates you from God. Meditate on God's Name. Embrace and practice Simran - remembrance of your True Identity. Worship and adore the Guru, the Perfect True Guru. All the errors of your past shall be washed away. By your great destiny, you shall know that bliss which passes all understanding. Har, Har, will become sweet to your mind. Servant Nanak proclaims that in this first round, the marriage ceremony has begun.*

*2. In the second round of the marriage ceremony, the Lord guides you to meet the True Guru - the Primal teacher within all. Filled with the awe of the Infinite, your ego dissolves away in the presence of the One who is forever pure. Sing His Praises and see the One in everyone. The Supreme Soul is the Master of the Universe. He fills everything, everywhere. He fills all spaces. Deep within us, and outside as well, there is only One. God's humble servants meet together and sing the songs of joy. Servant Nanak proclaims that in this second round, the music of the spheres resounds.*

*3. In the third round of the marriage ceremony our hearts are filled with Divine Love. By our great destiny we have met the humble Saints who love the Lord and we have found God. We have found the One and sing His praises. We speak the Gurbani. By our great destiny we have found the humble Saints and we speak the silent language of the Infinite. Har, Har, Har, vibrates and resounds within our hearts. Meditating on God, we have realized the great destiny inscribed upon our foreheads. Servant Nanak proclaims that in this third round, are hearts are filled with Divine Love of the One.*

*4. In the fourth round of the marriage ceremony we have found God and our minds are filled with peace. Living as Gurmukhs, we have met Him with simple ease. Our minds and bodies are full of sweet delight. Night and day we lovingly focus our awareness on the One. We have merged with the One and all our desires are fulfilled. The Naam resounds and reverberates within us and all around us. The Master, merges with His Divine Bride and her heart blossoms with His Holy Naam. Servant Nanak proclaims that in this fourth round, we have merged with the One in everyone.*

# CELESTIAL COMMUNICATION

### *By SS Gurukirn Kaur Khalsa*

*(From "Yogi Bhajan's Unique Contributions to Sikh Dharma")*

Children were always very special to Yogi Bhajan. He developed Celestial Communication to integrate them into the Gurdwara service. Just before "Song of the Khalsa," the children are invited to come up in front of the congregation and led by an adult or one of the older children, they interpret the meanings of the songs in gracefully choreographed arm and hand movements. Yogi Bhajan described it this way: "Celestial Communication makes a human very expressive and clear in thoughts. It's a science, not a joke. When you do it and encourage your children to do it, you are making them leaders of tomorrow. They can express themselves. They can create impact. They'll be free of the shyness with which you have suffered. So by participating like this today you have helped your children for tomorrow. If you do not prepare your children for tomorrow, you dare not have children. If you cannot prepare your children for tomorrow, it means you have not care."[64]

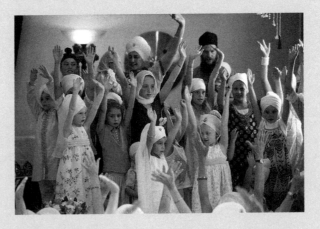

*Children doing Celestial Communication in the Española, New Mexico, Gurdwara*
*Photo by Gurumustuk Singh Khalsa*

---

[64] Khalsa Women's Training Camp, Gurdwara Lecture July 3, 1994

# The Celestial Communication Technique

*Yogi Bhajan, January 1, 1995*

Celestial Communication is for when you can't take care of your neurosis by any known method. There is no power greater than the power of the Word, and when the Word is performed through the body, the entire being is purified and relaxed.

If you are Christian, you are a Jew, you are a Moslem, you are a Hindu, you are a Sikh, you are a Buddhist, you are nobody, you are everybody -- science is science. Living in the 20th century and seeing people talking to themselves on the road, making a telephone call, drinking a cup of coffee, reading the newspaper, driving the car, and mostly being who they are -- and not being who they are -- something has to be given to mankind to excel, to come out of it without much cost. And that is what we have done.

We have transformed our songs to the strength of the communication of the Celestial Communication Technique, which is ours, which is our gift to the world through us and through our children to follow. It relaxes the brain through the nerve connections of the tips of the fingers, which are the main active parts and ingredients in this being. When the fingers move with the prana to communicate with music, this cantaloupe becomes the human brain and then tension of the neuro-pattern is restored into relaxed patterns of its own originality.

It's a very fantastic release. We practiced Celestial Communication at Khalsa Women's Training Camp, and this time every woman who went home to the city from the camp could not adjust at home. I understood. I never said that to you, but I knew that when the angels will reach and meet the mortal, it will be impossible to adjust. And I wanted to see that without doing a thing how much we can do and we did it. And we did a wonderful job.

Every human has the capacity of creative self and no person is weak or condemned in the eyes of God. Something, which I actually do not like, is when in my presence people put down other people. Reacting to people is not what you need. Directing people in their essence, and making them understand is a very simple known fact.

Physical relaxation is not as important as the neuro-system relaxation. That is why the Celestial Communication system will work wonders with all people from all religions and from all places. It is a methodology which will give everyone a tremendous amount of relief in their inner being.

Creativity, when combined with physical movement, psychological concentration, and meditation, is very helpful. It balances the human energy and it gives strength to the Radiant Body. This brings prosperity and success. People who against all odds, can smile, who against all provocation can peacefully talk, and against all obnoxiousness can behave beautifully, are bound to be very successful. There is no such thing as defeat for them.

# Children

Yogi Bhajan taught that through their prayer and meditation, parents can attract souls to this planet who will be saints, heroes, and givers, destined to uplift the consciousness of humanity. The frequency of the soul that enters the fetus on the 120th day of pregnancy matches the frequency of the consciousness of the mother. In order to support this most sacred time in the life of a mother, we hold a special 120th day celebration to honor the mother and prepare her consciousness to welcome the new soul. If for any reason the timing or environments are not right for the mother to be able to nurture a child, any time before the 120th day of her pregnancy she can have an abortion with a clear conscience because the soul has not yet entered her womb.

Yogi Bhajan used to call parents "pay rents." He said that children are a gift to us from God and that our only job is to nurture them, guide them, and teach them the values of *Khalsa*, conscious living. They are not "ours" to own or dominate with our egos. They are actually a sacred trust from the Infinite, and they belong to God, and like us, they will return to God when their time on this earth is finished.

# Education

## Miri Piri Academy—A Training Ground for the Spiritual Leaders and Peaceful Warriors of the Future

### By SS Sat Mander Kaur Khalsa

The Siri Singh Sahib, Yogi Bhajan, always taught with an eye on the future of humanity and the planet. He came to awaken us and prepare us for the transition into the Aquarian frequency of the coming Age. He began early on by reminding us that through the mothers' wombs would come the souls who would lead us into the future.

As the young adults of the late 1960s and early 1970s began to marry and raise families, he focused on the new generation who were growing up in our midst. The challenge was how to give them the foundation they needed to face the coming times and become spiritual leaders and global citizens of a transforming world.

In the early 1980s we began a school program in India for our children, which has evolved over the past twenty-five years to the point where we now have our own school near the city of Amritsar, India, called Miri Piri Academy.

Miri Piri refers to the balance of heavens and earth, spiritual and temporal realms. The goal of the Academy is to provide children with an education that focuses on the whole being: body, mind, and spirit. To this end, we have included training in Kundalini Yoga and yogic lifestyle teachings along with training in the values, spirit, and practice of Sikh Dharma, as well as academics, art, and physical education. The experience of attending a school far from their parents' home allows the children to develop self-mastery and self-reliance, an inner strength, which is brought out by the challenges, blessings, and opportunities of the environment. They bond with children from all over the globe and experience a culture that may be very different from that in which they began their lives, so their awareness of the diversity of the entire planet is increased. Being in Amritsar, the home of the Golden Temple, gives the children the opportunity to experience the divine vibration of this sacred spot, to dip in the healing nectar tank, or *sarovar,* of the Golden Temple, and to participate in many types of *seva*. Being in Amritsar also gives the children opportunities to study *Gurbani Kirtan* (devotional music), the science of *raag* with Indian masters of this ancient discipline, and to study *gatka*, a traditional martial art of the Sikhs.

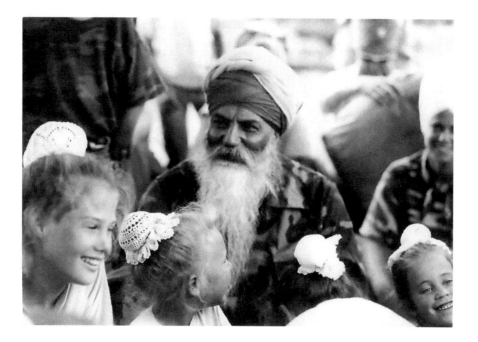

It was a monumental task to start a school, get the land, build the facilities, hire the teachers, and develop a network of financial, legal, and architectural wisdom in order to manifest this project. But somehow we did it, and today *Miri Piri Academy* educates over one hundred students from fifteen different countries.

To the Siri Singh Sahib, what was most important in the education of children was to build their character so that they could face their tomorrow with excellence and success. He wanted them to have the capacity to read the moment and adjust to any challenge. He wanted them to have deep self-mastery so they could manage a massive amount of information and yet keep their humanity intact. He taught them to face their destiny, to go the distance with purity of self, purity of thought, and purity of mission so each of them could excellently fulfill his or her own soul-contract with God.[65]

---

[65]  As described in the book: *Soul Contracts: How They Affect Our Life and Our Relationships,* by Linda Baker, 2003, ISBN-10: 0595267440.

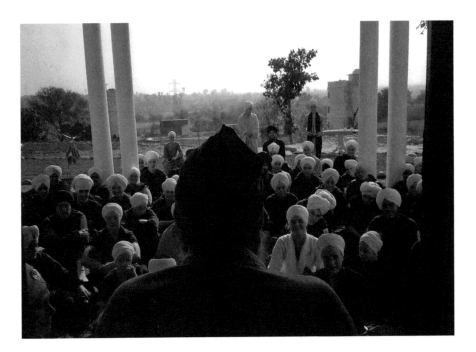

The Siri Singh Sahib addressed the students of MPA in Anandpur Sahib on January 3, 2001:

*"You must achieve three powers, and you will never be captured or conquered by anybody. It is purity of self, purity of thought, and purity of mission. If you can achieve these three powers combined together, their union will make you excellent…*

*"You are a human being par-excellence, born on your own longitude and latitude. That longitude and latitude will give you attitude, and then you have to look at the horizon of your extension where you want to be—and this is your power."*

# A Graduate's Personal Story

*Miri Piri Academy, India*
*By Guru Rattan Kaur Khalsa, Los Angeles, California*

As I arrived at the hot and stinky New Delhi airport in the early hours of the morning in India, I thought "What am I doing here?" As soon as we started on the eight-hour bus trip to Amritsar, I looked out the window at the dark shadows of India's night and realized this is where I would stay. I was on my way to school in the heart of every Sikh's heritage, Miri Piri Academy in the holy city of Amritsar.

I am a Mexican-American-Greek Sikh born into Sikhism because my parents became Sikhs in the 1970s because of the inspiration of 3HO and the Siri Singh Sahib. I knew I would go to school in India for at least a few years before I actually did in seventh grade, because my sister, who is nine years older than I, had been to a few of the previous schools in India. I went to grade school in Los Angeles, California, where I was born and now I am going to college there, but these schools will never compare with the life I had at MPA.

Before I left home, all my friends told me that I wouldn't be able to handle going to MPA because it was a very strict military-like academy, and we didn't see our parents for nine months per year unless they came to visit. But as I learned, being away from my parents for so long with all the discipline that was brought upon us helped me grow into a stronger individual. I have found, as I'm sure many others at MPA have, that discipline is the best way to achieve happiness. Very rarely was someone unhappy at MPA.

MPA students live in dorms so we learn to respect people's space and at the same time become close and trusting. We shared everything at MPA—our rooms, our food, our belongings, and our thoughts. We all became close because we all were experiencing the same day-to-day doings. I understand that now they are slowly expanding the capacity of the school, adding second stories and more dorm rooms. I hope that in spite of an increase in the number of students, they will still be able to enjoy the same cozy familiarity that we all had when I was there.

At MPA we learned to be teachers, not followers. We were given the privilege in grade 11 to become Certified Kundalini Yoga Teachers. With this training we could help others become stronger. Kundalini Yoga was a big part of our daily lifestyle. We would have at least one class a day so we grew not only to love it, but embrace the Siri Singh Sahib's teachings so that later as teachers, we could share what we had learned.

MPA students have vigorous, independent minds because of MPA's disciplined regimen, curriculum, and staff. I have become the strong-minded person I am today because of what Miri Piri Academy overall has taught me. I love and miss MPA and hope to one day send my children there.

To learn more about Miri Piri Academy, visit www.miripiriacademy.org.

# Chapter Eleven

# Akal-Deathlessness

☬

# MY PERSONAL EXPERIENCES WITH DEATH

## The Big Sleep (not the movie)[66]
..................................................................................................................

*By MSS Shakti Parwha Kaur Khalsa*

*"Everyone wants to go to heaven, but nobody wants to die."*

That was a favorite quote back in the early days of 3HO. Surprisingly, some of the most inspiring, uplifting, and amazing experiences in my adult life have come when I was in the presence of death.

However, probably because my father committed suicide when I was 13, for many years I blotted out thoughts about death. As far as I was concerned, death was just a permanent, dreamless sleep. I had never

---
66 Reprinted from Aquarian Times.

attended a funeral until 1969 when I went with Yogi Bhajan to a memorial service for Peter the Hermit, a well-known metaphysical teacher whom we had met a few weeks earlier at his Hollywood Hills home. At that meeting, I remember Yogiji saying to Peter, "It's time to change your shirt." I didn't realize then what he meant was that it was Peter's time to "go."

When "the Yogi" spoke about death at the funeral, it was in glowing, inspiring terms from an understanding I'd never heard before. The concept of being "called Home" to reunite with your Creator, the Source of all life, when your allotment of breaths for this lifetime has been used up was new to me.

# Touching a Corpse

Early in the 1970s, an infant in our community died of SIDS (Sudden Infant Death Syndrome). I felt obliged to go to the mortuary and be there with the father and the Sikh minister who was preparing the body for cremation[67] according to Sikh tradition. I was not thrilled being in a funeral parlor, and certainly had no intention of participating in the Sikh rite of bathing the body in yogurt before cremation. Yet, as the minister was reciting *Japji Sahib* and beginning to apply the yogurt to the tiny body, I could see another pair of hands was needed. I stepped up, and to my amazement, as I grasped one tiny baby leg for support, it felt as if I were holding a rubber doll, and even more amazing, as I touched this corpse (yes, I was holding a dead body), I felt the outer corners of my mouth involuntarily curling up into a blissful smile. I experienced a sense of total tranquility, peace, and joy. God was surely close to Earth that day, collecting the innocent soul who had been called Home.

# The Power of Akaal

I think one of the most painful things about the death of someone close is the feeling of helplessness, that there's nothing you can do. That's why I so much appreciate the Sikh Dharma (and yogic) tradition of chanting *Akaal* when someone dies.

When my mother died at the age of 94, it was a great consolation for me to be able to stand next to her hospital bed with four Sikh women friends chanting *Akaal*. As I looked at her lifeless body, I knew for sure my mother wasn't there; it was just an empty shell, and I was grateful I could help her soul on its journey.

My son died suddenly and unexpectedly of a heart attack in 1998, at the age of 49. Again, I experienced the incredible blessing of being part of this Sikh Dharma family. Members of the community rallied around and virtually cushioned me through all the funeral preparations. Knowing death to be a journey home, I ordered "Bon Voyage" balloons. I knew it had to be a celebration. James was finally free of the *karma* of this incarnation. As the casket was about to be consigned to the flames of the crematorium, about fifty of us chanted *Akaal, Akaal, Akaal*, over and over, led by the Siri Singh Sahib, whose voice resonated with

---

[67] Cremation of the physical body releases the *tattvas*, or elements which comprise the physical body, and breaks the magnetic attachment to the earth's energy field, thus releasing the soul and subtle bodies to transition more easily to the higher dimensions.

such power and passion, it was as if thousands upon thousands of beings were chanting with us, joining in and echoing the call to deathlessness. For me, that day was exhilarating and uplifting, almost transcendental.

The chanting of *Akaal* creates a vibratory frequency that assists the departing soul, carried by the subtle body, on its journey through the ethers to final liberation. The subtle body is one of our ten energetic bodies. (It represents calmness, mastery, and subtlety.)

For several weeks I felt calm, apparently "normal," feeling and thinking I was fine. I didn't realize that I was actually in a state of shock. Then to my surprise, James' death hit me, and I started experiencing the textbook stages of mourning. I had thought that since I understood the spiritual meaning of death, I assumed that I would just accept my son's departure without emotion. Well, I had forgotten what Yogi Bhajan had taught me about *being human* when Bhai Sahib Dayal Singh died in an automobile accident at the age of 21.[68] Here's that story.

# The "Accident"

In 1975, a *Yatra* (pilgrimage) to India was planned, and Bhai Sahib was eager to go. He went to the Siri Singh Sahib to ask permission. The Siri Singh Sahib told him that yes, he could go to India, but he should not drive. Unfortunately, Bhai Sahib didn't mention that he didn't have enough money to pay for the flight from Los Angeles to New York, the main departure point for the group. I suppose he interpreted the "don't drive" to mean only that he shouldn't be behind the wheel, rather than not being in a car at all. And so, Bhai Sahib Ji took off for New York as a passenger in someone else's car.

Early in the morning, passing through Indiana, the car in which he was a passenger crashed, and he was thrown out of the car and killed instantly. Others in the car were severely injured. Interestingly enough, before leaving Los Angeles, he had given away most of his possessions, and organized his few remaining belongings in his room at Adi Shakti Ashram.

# Should Yogis Mourn?

The Siri Singh Sahib was flying back to Los Angeles from a lecture tour when I got a phone call from his Chief of Staff, Nirinjan Kaur, telling me that Bhai Sahib Dayal Singh had been killed. So, when the Siri Singh Sahib arrived at Guru Ram Das Ashram, it was my unhappy task to tell him what had happened.

He, members of his staff, and I sat in the living room of Guru Ram Das Ashram, talking about the "accident." I didn't want anyone to see me crying, so I kept going into the bathroom to splash cold water on my face and try to compose myself. After about four such trips, Yogiji said, "What are you doing?" I said, "I know yogis are not supposed to be emotional and cry." He looked at me as if I were crazy, and said, "Aren't you human?" Thus I learned that even though we know what death really means, we still have a legitimate human right— if not a need—to experience sorrow for our loss.

---

[68]  More about Bhai Sahib Dyal Singh on page 139

Later on, I remember him saying, with tears rolling down his cheeks, that God had picked the most beautiful flower from his garden. He also said that when the car went off the road, Bhai Sahib Dayal Singh was not in his body; he was already at the Golden Temple with all the Gurus and in complete bliss.

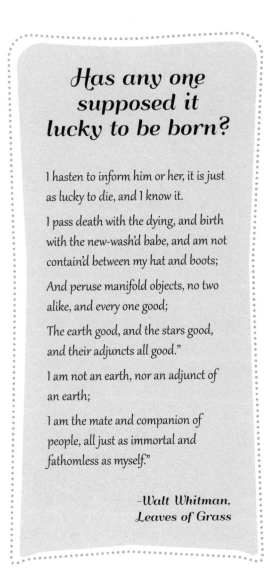

*Has any one supposed it lucky to be born?*

*I hasten to inform him or her, it is just as lucky to die, and I know it.*

*I pass death with the dying, and birth with the new-wash'd babe, and am not contain'd between my hat and boots;*

*And peruse manifold objects, no two alike, and every one good;*

*The earth good, and the stars good, and their adjuncts all good."*

*I am not an earth, nor an adjunct of an earth;*

*I am the mate and companion of people, all just as immortal and fathomless as myself."*

*-Walt Whitman,*
*Leaves of Grass*

# Death and Taxes

They say two things are inevitable—death and taxes. We are all born to die. That's a fact. Well, that being the case, it seems advisable to get all our accounts in order, save all our receipts, and be ready for the examiner to see what *karma* is left to pay. Yet, it is only the body that dies when the soul departs. The soul is immortal and indestructible. Even though air is left in the body, it is *prana*—the divine life force that is withdrawn and, if we are ready, returns directly to God, without having to come back into another human form. All things come from God, and all things (including us) shall return to God, the source of all life. The trick is to die consciously. That's what yogis have done while still in the body. They tell us that death is simply a return to the Source. It is nothing to fear. Many of us work to achieve that state of yoga, or Divine Union, while still alive, so that when it is finally time to leave behind this rented vehicle, we shall have a swift, smooth, direct, non-stop journey Home. Meanwhile, we do trial runs, field trips—called meditation.

# Constant Remembrance of Death

The official Sikh code of conduct, a blueprint for living on this spiritual path, is called the *Rehit Maryada*, which means "constant remembrance of death." When I first heard about this, I thought it sounded really morbid, but the more I thought about it, the more it made sense.

Have you seen movies where the hero (or heroine) is told that he/she only has six months to live? Usually a major transformation of character happens at that point.

What would you do? How would you live your life? In Charles Dickens' *A Christmas Carol*, the meanest of the mean, Mr. Ebenezer Scrooge, definitely changes his attitude and actions after he's shown what legacy he would leave if he continued his selfish and stingy ways!

Knowing that each inhalation could be our last provides a practical touchstone, a perspective from which to assess all our words and actions. Death becomes a constant presence. And you know what? It's not morbid at all. In fact, it's exhilarating!

# Live Long and Prosper

Ancient wisdom states that whenever a baby is born, the life span is already predetermined, not by the number of years he or she will live, but by the number of breaths allotted. When you've used up your ration of *prana*, the incoming life breath, your time on this planet is over. The *prana* is withdrawn, and we call it Death. Accidents or illness are only *apparent* causes of death; we simply die when there is no more *prana* in the body. So, the slower and deeper you breathe, the longer you'll live. (Which makes sense because you'll be calmer and relaxed, putting less wear and tear on the body, and that would contribute to your general health and enjoyment of longevity.)

# What Happens After Death?

As a young man, Yogi Bhajan took a tourist party to a special shrine in the Himalayas. Hot and thirsty after the long climb, he drank a large glass of ice-cold water and passed out cold. After 45 minutes of no life signs, he was declared dead. "Miraculously"—by the grace of God—he revived. Afterward he recalled the choice he had been given: On the right side of a fork in the road, he saw a warm and welcoming tavern with friends and relatives beckoning him to enter. On the left was a cold and snowy path. Fortunately for us, he chose neither, and came back into his body to serve humanity for many more years. When our time comes, he advises, "Choose the snowy path." That's the one that leads to liberation. He has also said that, as our Spiritual Teacher, he will be there to guide us.

Meanwhile, as we journey through time and space in these physical vehicles, may we use our precious breath to make this a better world for our having lived and breathed here!

# Coming and Going – The Big Picture

### By SS Sat Mander Kaur Khalsa

In most of the eastern traditions, including Sikh Dharma, it is understood that human life is a temporary state, something we experience between birth and death. But "we" (meaning our spirit or soul—within the essence of our being) are already immortal, undying, a permanent part of the Infinite or God. We just don't know it, until or unless we make a conscious effort to realize our True identity. It is only in this human incarnation, living in a finite body, with a finite ego, that we can experience our Infinite Identity.

We evolve through the experience of many lifetimes to reach the point where we are ready to take advantage of this potential. Once it is experienced, we will be eager to share it so others can have the same experience.

Ordinarily, we spend our time on Earth living our *karma*, gradually learning the life lessons we need in order to progress in our evolution of awareness and consciousness. When we choose to live a dharma, a path of spiritual consciousness, we can stop the chain of action–reaction and consciously enter the flow of the entire creation, merging finite and infinite aspects of our being. It takes discipline and practice along with commitment to the process, but the spiritual technology of a dharma, or spiritual path, is intended to lead us to this ultimate human potential. The teachings and technology of Sikh Dharma are powerful tools to guide us to our highest consciousness, leading us to the experience of our true, Infinite identity.

With this perspective, we see the "end" of this lifetime as the beginning of whatever the next stage of evolution brings. It is a transition we all shall make. It can be transformational for ourselves and for those who love us, especially if we are able to approach it without fear.

# Death: Philosophically Speaking

### By MSS Shakti Parwha Kaur Khalsa

*"All things come from God and all things shall return to God."*[69] *(including us)*

We don't die because of accident, illness, or old age. We are pronounced dead only when there is no more breath, no more *prana* in us.

When all the breaths we were allotted for this lifetime have been used up, the Creator, the One God who breathes in each of us, withdraws that breath of life from the physical body, and the soul, transported by the subtle body, leaves the physical body.

Ideally, at the moment of death, we remember to chant God's Name, because usually whatever thought, word, or idea (i.e., vibratory frequency) is in our mind at the moment of death determines where our soul is headed: into another incarnation, or back Home to God. That's one reason why developing the habit of chanting God's Name now, while we are alive, is such a valuable practice.

We chant *Akaal* when someone dies in order to assist the soul in leaving the Earth's atmosphere, or electromagnetic field, so it can go directly to reach the ultimate state of Deathlessness. (*Kaal* means death, *Akaal* means deathless.) Once *Akaal Purkh* is reached, the soul doesn't have to reincarnate again.

Remember, the body isn't you, the mind isn't you. Those are just convenient vehicles. They are not the real you! You are a divine, immortal being, temporarily here on Earth to experience God's creation and to learn to be human. Your true identity is *Sat Nam* – which is also God's Name.

# *In Memoriam*

Most people leave it to others, but not the Siri Singh Sahib! Several years before his death in 2004, he composed his own epitaph. He commissioned Amrit Singh Khalsa to build the gray granite marker at the Ranch in Española, New Mexico, where the Siri Singh Sahib lived for over twenty-five years. The marker stands exactly six feet-two inches tall and three feet wide. The words he chose to be chiseled in the stone surely express the essence of his life and how he experienced Death: becoming One with God.

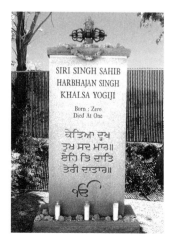

Guru Simran Kaur Khalsa, the faithful caretaker of the Ranch property for many years, told me how the Siri Singh Sahib planned this remarkable stone:

---

[69] From a song composed at Khalsa Women's Training Camp based on Yogi Bhajan's teachings.

· · · · · · · · · · · · · · · · · · · · · · · · · · · · · · · · · · · · · · · · · · · · · · · · · · · · · · · · · · · · · · · · · · · · · · · · · · · · ·

*"Some people asked the Siri Singh Sahib, 'Sir, we know who you are; at least we know you in person. But what about the children who are still to be born in the future and the yoga students who haven't met you? How can they understand who you are?'"*

His directions to Amrit Singh Khalsa were, *"Take a stone as tall as I am and on the front you write: Born Zero, Died at One."*

· · · · · · · · · · · · · · · · · · · · · · · · · · · · · · · · · · · · · · · · · · · · · · · · · · · · · · · · · · · · · · · · · · · · · · · · · · · · ·

He said that people might not understand these words now, but future generations will.

· · · · · · · · · · · · · · · · · · · · · · · · · · · · · · · · · · · · · · · · · · · · · · · · · · · · · · · · · · · · · · · · · · · · · · · · · · · · ·

*"Then you write the line from the 25th pauri (of Japji Sahib):* **Ketia dukh bukh sad mar, eh bee dat teree daataar** *(*'Whatever pain and suffering come to me, these too are Your blessings, O Lord')*. When they meditate on this, they will understand the motto I lived by. And on the back write the words to the 'Song of the Khalsa.'"*[70].

· · · · · · · · · · · · · · · · · · · · · · · · · · · · · · · · · · · · · · · · · · · · · · · · · · · · · · · · · · · · · · · · · · · · · · · · · · · · ·

---

[70]  See page 151

# Epilogue

## OUR SPIRITUAL FUTURE[71]

*by Yogi Bhajan*


*We are building a nation, sovereign and spiritual.*
*We are building a tradition*
*And we are wearing a beautiful hand woven yarmulke,*
*Which we tie every day.*


*And we are pretending and projecting*
*That we are aware of the Christ Consciousness,*
*And we know, through wisdom, the Buddhi,*
*And we know, through humility, the Islam,*
*And we seek, as a Sikh, the Truth.*


*So we are a multiple combination of everything which ever existed,*
*Because we have a focus:*
*And our focus is the Reality of God*
*In the Totality of Man.*


*Siri Singh Sahib Bhai Sahib*
*Harbhajan Singh Khalsa Yogiji, April 9, 1980*

---

[71] Reprinted with permission from The Game of Love: Poems of Consciousness By Yogi Bhajan

# "Ocean of Love" by Kabir

Kabir was a Hindu weaver by profession yet he ranks as one of the world's greatest poets. He is one of the enlightened *Bhagats* (poets) included in the *Siri Guru Granth Sahib*. Their words ring true because they are based upon each author's personal experience of Divine Union with God, and the wisdom and understanding gained in that blissful state. In his writings, Kabir made a serious effort to unite Muslims and Hindus.

*"I have found something,*
*Something rare have I found;*
*Its value none can assess.*

*It has no color, it is One,*
*Indivisible and everlasting*
*Untouched by the waves of change,*
*It fills each and every vessel.*

*It has no weight, it has no price;*
*Beyond the bounds of measurement,*
*It cannot be counted,*
*And through erudition*
*It cannot be known.*
*It is neither heavy nor light,*
*No touchstone can assay its worth.*

*I dwell in it, it dwells in me,*
*We are One,*
*Like water mixed with water.*
*He who knows it,*
*Will never die;*
*He who knows it not,*
*Dies again and again.*

*Kabir, the Lord's slave, has discovered*
*An ocean filled with the nectar of love;*
*But I find no one disposed to taste it.*
*When men do not believe my words,*
*Words from my own experience,*
*What else can I say to convince them?"*

# Appendix

## The Sikh Calendar

### Sikh Dharma Holidays

Sikh Holy Days are called *Gurpurbs*. These holidays are sacred occasions, joyously (sacred doesn't mean somber!) and gratefully celebrated in honor, remembrance, and appreciation of people and events that shaped the evolution of Sikh Dharma from its beginnings.

The *Gurdwara* is the focal point of all *Gurpurbs*. *Langar* and *Gurbani Kirtan* are welcome components of all Sikh holidays. We love to sing, and we love to feed people.

### Birthdays and Other Occasions

There are many, many notable occasions Sikhs have reason to value and acknowledge, such as the birthdays and dates of installation (*Guru Gaddi*) of the Gurus (as well as the birthdays and deaths of the four sons of Guru Gobind Singh who gave their lives for their faith). However, following are the major holidays that are emphasized:

# Guru Gaddee Day

Guru Gaddee Day is the celebration of the installation in 1708 of the *Siri Guru Granth Sahib* as the final and only living Guru of all Sikhs by Guru Gobind Singh. This historic occasion is celebrated with what is called a *Jaloose*, a procession in which the *Siri Guru Granth Sahib* is carried in regal splendor on a *palki sahib* (platform) on the shoulders of members of the *sangat* (congregation). We chant as we walk to the destination Gurdwara, where, of course, there will be music and *langar.*

# Guru Ram Das's Birthday

From all over the world, thousands of devotees flock to Amritsar, India, every year to celebrate the Fourth Guru's birthday. It was there that Guru Ram Das founded the exquisite and incomparable Golden Temple.

The Siri Singh Sahib, Bhai Sahib Harbhajan Singh Khalsa Yogiji, introduced Westerners to Guru Ram Das and the Sikh way of life. At his suggestion, we celebrate the birthday of Guru Ram Das (with whom he had a transformative experience when he was nine years old) by chanting *Dhan Dhan Ram Das Gur* [72] for two and a half hours.

In many Sikh Dharma communities, on the elelven days leading up to the birthday of Guru Ram Das, we get together for a cozy evening at different community members' homes to chant *Dhan Dhan Ram Das Gur* and enjoy *langar.*

# Guru Nanak's Birthday

This usually falls sometime in November and one way we celebrate is with continuous recitations of *Japji Sahib*—and of course, a special Gurdwara.

# Guru Gobind Singh's Birthday

*Incorporating 31 minutes of bowing to Jaap Sahib* [73] *during early morning sadhana is a great way to celebrate the Tenth Guru's birthday in January! What we are bowing to is really our own highest consciousness.*

---

[72]  Dhan Dhan Ram Das Gur, see page 55

[73]  Ragi Sat Nam Singh Sethi's CD is ideal for this.

# Yogi Bhajan's Birthday

Many years ago, when we were determined to celebrate the Siri Singh Sahib's (Yogi Bhajan's) birthday, he asked us to use it as a Day of Prayer for Peace. So we celebrate August 26th every year with 11 minutes of worldwide simultaneous chanting of *Guru Guru Wahe Guru.*[74] *This is preceded—or followed—by two and a half hours of chanting Long Ek Ong Kar's,*[75] depending on the local time zone.

(See *Frequently Chanted Mantras and Shabds* in the Appendix for the words of the shabds and an English translation.)

---

[74] Guru Guru Wahe Guru, see page 56
[75] Long Ek Ong Kar's, see page 54

# *Dateline of Sikh Dharma History-Making Events*

1.  January 5, 1969: Yogi Bhajan gives his first public lecture in the U.S.A.

2.  April 1970: First Americans take formal vows as Sikhs.

3.  December 1970: Yogi Bhajan takes eighty-four Kundalini Yoga students on Yatra[76] to India; many take Amrit at the Akal Takhat.

4.  March 3, 1971: First ever title of "Siri Singh Sahib" is bestowed on Yogi Bhajan at the Akal Takhat in Amritsar.

5.  March 8, 1971: Letter issued by the SGPC[77] gives the Siri Singh Sahib authority to establish an ordained Ministry in the West, perform marriages, administer final rites, and administer Amrit according to Sikh tradition.

6.  1971: First American-English translation of Sikh prayers (*Peace Lagoon*) is published.

7.  December 23, 1971: Yogi Bhajan buys the property at 1620 Preuss Road in Los Angeles to be Guru Ram Das Ashram.

8.  January 1972: First Western-born Sikhs ordained as Ministers by the Siri Singh Sahib.

9.  June 23, 1972: First "Sikh Dharma" flag unfurled at the Mendocino, California, Summer Solstice Camp. First women ordained as Sikh Dharma Ministers.

10. April 10, 1973: Articles of Incorporation for "Sikh Dharma Brotherhood" endorsed by the Secretary of State of California as an official religious organization. This name was later changed legally to "Sikh Dharma International."

11. June 1973: First title of "Bhai Sahib" given by the Siri Singh Sahib to the Head *Granthi* (Dayal Singh Khalsa).

12. October 24, 1974: Khalsa Council established as Chief Administrative Body of Sikh Dharma of the Western Hemisphere.

---

[76]  pilgrimage
[77]  Shromani Gurdwara Prabhandak Committee

# Glossary

## A

**Adi Granth** – Original collection of sacred writings of the first five Sikh Gurus and other Hindu, Muslim and Sufi saints, completed in 1604 by Guru Arjan.

 **Adi Shakti** (also **Khanda**) – Primal creative feminine power. Preeminent Sikh insignia formed by a combination of a chakra, a khanda, and two kirpans.

**Akal** or **Akaal** – Undying; deathless; beyond death. This mantra is chanted upon a person's death to assist the departing soul on its journey home to God.

**Akhand Path** – Continuous unbroken reading (aloud) of the entire *Siri Guru Granth Sahib*. Traditionally, this takes 48 hours in the original *Gurmukhi*. It takes 72 hours in English.

**Amrit – Nectar.** The transformed water used in the baptismal ceremony known as the *Amrit Sanchar*.

**Amrit Dhari** – Sikh who has taken Amrit to become Khalsa. "Dhari" means "practitioner" or "endowed with" (lit. having taken the Amrit).

**Amrit Sanchar** – Baptismal ceremony instituted in 1699 by Guru Gobind Singh.

**Amrit Vela** – Period three hours before sunrise, ideal for meditation.

**Anand Sahib** – Song of Bliss, written by Guru Amar Das. One of the Banis, portions of which are played in Gurdwara.

**Ang Sang Wahe Guru** – Pronounced "ung sung waa-hay gu-roo." "In every part of my being is the ecstasy of God's wonder." "God is in every part of me." "God and me are One."

**Ardas** – Traditional Sikh prayer, usually recited before reading of Hukam.

**Aura** – Electromagnetic field that surrounds each person.

**Baba Buddha or Bhai Buddha** – Baba Buddha was a most respected saint. He occupies a unique position in Sikh history. He applied the mark of guruship to five Gurus, saw seven Gurus, and remained in close association with first six Sikh Gurus from 1521 to 1628 for over one hundred years. He was the first priest of *Harimandir Sahib*, and laid the foundations of most of the holy buildings at Amritsar.

**Baisakhi** – A spring holiday which occurs during mid-April every year and traditionally, in the Punjab, concurs with the first harvesting of the crops for the year. So, historically, it has been a very joyous occasion and a time for celebration. It also commemorates the founding of the Khalsa by Guru Gobind Singh in 1699.

## B

**Bana** – Distinctive Sikh clothing including a turban.

**Bani** – Words, usually in verse.

**Banis** – Special Sikh prayers, composed in a sound current tuned for raising human consciousness.

**Bhagat** – Poet or minstrel. The word Bhagat comes from the Sanskrit word Bhakti, which means lover of God. The poems of fifteen such saints who were not Sikh Gurus, but simply enlightened followers of the path of devotion and surrender, are included in the *Siri Guru Granth Sahib.*

**Bhai Gurdas** – A much-honored Sikh scholar, missionary, and literary master. The nephew of Guru Amar Das, the third Sikh Guru, he was a leading figure in Sikh history who enjoyed the company of Guru Arjan, the fifth Sikh Guru. Under Guru Arjan's supervision, he inscribed the Adi Granth, the first copy of the Guru Granth Sahib.

**Bhakti** – 1) Devotion to God. 2) Devotee; "Lover of God" (Sanskrit).

# C

**Chakra** – 1) A steel ring worn around turban. One of the central elements of the Adi Shakti insignia—a circle designating infinity. 2) In yogic terms, one of the energy Centers of the body.

**Chauri** – The Chauri Sahib is a decorated whisk, which is waved gently over the Guru Granth Sahib as a mark of sovereignty and honor.

**Chola** – Simple long cotton or silk shirt.

**Chuni** – Sheer scarf worn by Sikh women draped over the turban.

**Churidars** – Long pants tapered from the knees down to fit snugly at ankles.

**Cummerbund** – Waist sash.

# D

**Darbar** – The court of the Guru.

**Darshan** – Blessing of seeing or being seen by a holy person.

**Dasvandh** – Tithe one-tenth of one's earnings.

**Dharma** – Spiritual way of life, including truth, contentment, compassion, and purity, leading to union with the Infinite Creator.

**Diwali** – The joyous Hindu Festival of Lights celebrated in November. Also known as Bandi Chor, it commemorates Guru Hargobind's release from Gwalior Fort prison around 1617.

# F

**Five K's** or **Five Kakars** – Five articles of dress worn by Amrit Dhari Sikhs, which identify the wearer as Khalsa. Originally given by Guru Gobind Singh during the Baisakhi ceremony in 1699, they are kachhera, kanga, kara, kesh, and kirpan.

# G

**Gaddee** – Throne.

**Granthi** – Minister. One who attends the Guru. One who directly serves the *Siri Guru Granth Sahib* in the Gurdwaras.

**Gunas** – Three qualities inherent in every living being: *Rajas* (energetic/fiery/outgoing/assertive); *Tamas* (lethargy, holding on to the status quo); *Sattva* (balance/equilibrium).

**Gurbani** – The Guru's word, compositions in *naad*; a perfect combination of sounds related to all the five elements in complete balance.

**Gurdwara** – Literally, "the Gate of the Guru." A sanctified place where the *Siri Guru Granth Sahib* is installed. Also a Sikh worship service held in the Gurdwara. It can be in an elaborate temple or in someone's living room, which has been cleared of furniture. Clean white sheets cover the floor, and the *Siri Guru Granth Sahib* is placed on a throne, an elevated platform, known as the Paulki Sahib.

**Gurmukhi** – The simplified phonetic alphabet codified by Guru Angad, the second Sikh Guru. Literally, "from the mouth of the Guru," the script used for writing and transcribing the biography and hymns of the Sikh Gurus.

**Gurprashad** – Sweet pudding made from wheat flour, water, ghee (clarified butter), and honey or sugar. It is served to all after the Hukam is read in the Gurdwara. (Literally: Gift of the Guru.)

**Gurpurb** – Sikh holiday.

**Guru** – One who takes you from darkness to light. Title applied to Nanak and his nine successors. The common term for the *Siri Guru Granth Sahib.*

**Guru ka Langar** – Community vegetarian meal, prayerfully prepared and served to all equally.

# H

**Harimandir Sahib** – Temple of God, holiest sanctuary of the Sikhs. Founded in 1601 by Guru Arjan in Amritsar, India. Commonly called the Golden Temple.

**Householder** – A person who works and lives in the everyday world. Not a recluse.

**Hukam** – Divine Will of God. The Guru's "order," a passage meditatively taken at random from the *Siri Guru Granth Granth* and read out loud to the congregation in the Gurdwara ceremony.

# I

 **Ik Ongkar** (also **Ek Ong Kar**) – All is One, One Creator created creation. First phrase and essence of the *Siri Guru Granth Sahib.* One of most common symbols of Sikhism. *Ek Ong Kaar*: One Creator created this Creation: There is only ONE. The visible and the invisible flow into one another through time and beyond time.

# J

**Japa** – Repeated recitation (of God's Name). Verbal recitation or chanting aloud.

**Joora** – Rishi knot. Hair coiled on top of the head and held in place with the kanga (wooden comb).

# K

**Kachhera (Katchera)** – Loose cotton under-shorts. One of the five K's.

**Kali Yug** – The Age of Darkness, lasting 432,000 years.

**Kanga** – Wooden comb. One of the five K's.

**Kara** – Steel or iron bracelet. One of the five K's.

**Karma** – Cosmic law of action and reaction, cause and effect ("As you sow, so shall you reap").

**Kaur** – Princess; last name for Sikh women, given by Guru Gobind Singh.

**Kesh** – Uncut hair. One of the five K's.

**Khalsa** – Pure one. Baptized Sikh. One who has received the Guru's Amrit.

**Khanda** – Double-edged sword, part of the Adi Shakti insignia. Used to stir the Amrit in the Amrit Sanchar ceremony.

**Kirpan** – Short curved sword. One of the five K's.

**Kirtan** (also **Gurbani Kirtan**) – Singing of the sacred hymns of the Guru.

# L

**Langar** – Meal offered to everyone. Common, free kitchen.

# M

**Mantra** – Sound current; mantric – having sound current

**Maya** – The phenomenal, measurable world; anything with a beginning and an end, usually defined as "illusion" since it is finite, not permanent, not Infinite.

**Missal** – A small working team that performs a particular service such as langar preparation or cleaning the Gurdwara.

# N

**Naad** – The inner sound current, tuned for raising human consciousness. Inner power and strength of sound.

**Nagara** – A very large kettledrum used in battle and in the Gurdwara.

**Nam Simran** – Meditation on the Name of God. Remembrance of one's own Infinite Identity.

**Nine Treasures** – Precious metals; gems and jewels; delicious foods; training in the use of arms; beautiful clothing and various staples; trade in gold; trade in gems; mastery of fine arts; and all kinds of riches.

**Nitnem Banis** – Daily prayers. Daily recitation of Sikh prayers.

# P

**Panj Piaray** – Five Beloved Ones. The original five Sikhs baptized by Guru Gobind Singh, becoming the first Khalsa at the Baisakhi ceremony in 1699.

**Panth** – The Sikh Community worldwide. Spiritual family. The global family of all Sikhs.

**Patka** – Small topknot style turban worn by young boys.

**Pauri** – Section, stanza or verse, as in a poem.

**Persian Wheel** – A water wheel with a number of blades, buckets, or pots arranged on the outside rim forming the driving surface.

**Pothi** – Traveling composition book, carried by Guru Nanak. Became the basis for the *Siri Guru Granth Sahib*.

**Prana** – Breath of Life. Incoming Breath. God's gift of life.

**Prashad** – Blessing or "gift" in the form of a sweet pudding given to congregants after a Gurdwara service (see Gurprashad). Pudding made of ghee, whole-wheat flour, and honey; cooked while *Japji* is being recited.

# R

**Raag** – Literally "color" or "mood." In Indian music, a series of five or more musical notes upon which a melody is founded. In the Indian musical tradition, ragas are played at different times of the day. Classic traditional Indian musical tonal patterns.

**Ragis** – Musicians who sing and play sacred Sikh music.

**Raj Yoga** – Royal path of Yoga (outlined in Patanjali's Sutras).

**Ramalas** – Elegant decorative fabric used to clothe the *Siri Guru Granth Sahib*.

**Rehit Maryada** – "Constant remembrance of death." Sikh code of conduct.

# S

**Sadh Sangat** – Gathering of the Holy (disciplined ones). Divine congregation.

**Sadhana** – Daily spiritual discipline. For Sikhs the daily practice of rising early, meditating and praising God's Name.

**Sahib** – Term of respect, usually affixed at end of man's name. It also means "grace" (feminine – **Sahiba**).

**Sangat** – Congregation. Those who do sadhana. The company of people of Truth.

**Sat Nam** – God's Identity is Truth. Truth is our Identity.

**Seva** – Selfless service.

**Shabd** – Sound current, but not just any sound. It is a sound vibration that cuts away the ego that obstructs the truth and prevents us from perceiving and acting from our authentic Self; vibratory frequency; also a selection from the *Siri Guru Granth Sahib* put to music.

**Shabd Guru** – A quantum technology of sound which directly alters our consciousness through the power of the Naad. Sound which teaches from within. The Word of God, articulated through the instrument of the Guru. The Guru or teacher in the form of the sound current contained in the *Siri Guru Granth Sahib*.

**Shakti** – God's power in manifestation. The feminine, creative aspect of God.

**Shakti Pad** – The stage in one's spiritual growth when the ego takes over.

**Shasters** – Swords or weapons in general.

**Shastra** – A scripture containing specific knowledge.

**Siddhi** – Yogic power.

**Sikh** – A student of Truth.

**Sikh Dharma** – Spiritual way of life based upon the teachings of the Ten Sikh Gurus and the *Siri Guru Granth Sahib*.

**Singh** – Lion; last name for Sikh men, given by the Tenth Guru.

**Siri** – Great.

**Siri Guru Granth Sahib** – The living Guru of the Sikhs. A universal technology for transformation of consciousness. It is quite literally the embodiment of the intrinsic wisdom of the Shabd Guru.

**Siri Singh Sahib** – Ministerial title as Chief Religious and Administrative Authority for Sikh Dharma of the Western Hemisphere bestowed upon Harbhajan Singh Khalsa Yogiji at the Akal Takhat by Sant Chanan Singh, in 1971. There had been no predecessors and are never to be any successors to this title.

**Sutras** – Lines or sections of a sacred poem.

# T

**Takhat** – Undying Throne; seat of religious authority. Guru Gobind Singh established Four Takhats (although some copies of the Ardas say there are five):

**Akal Takhat** in Amritsar (adjacent to the Golden Temple)

**Sri Takhat Keshgarh Sahib** in Anandpur Sahib (the city that Guru Gobind Singh founded and where he resided)

**Takhat Sachkhand** in Hazoor Sahib (the place where Guru Gobind Singh breathed his final breath)

**Sri Harimandir Takhat** in Patna (the birthplace of Guru Gobind Singh)

**Tattwas** – The five elements: earth, water, fire, air and ether.

**Ten Gurus** – The founder of the Sikh religion and his nine successors: 1) Guru Nanak; 2) Guru Angad; 3) Guru Amar Das; 4) Guru Ram Das; 5) Guru Arjan; 6) Guru Hargobind; 7) Guru Har Rai; 8) Guru Harkrishan; 9) Guru Tegh Bahadur; 10) Guru Gobind Singh.

**Turban** – A long piece of cloth wrapped around the head. Traditional article of dress for Sikhs. A regal crown of consciousness.

# W

**Wahe Guru** – Wondrous. Indescribable. Ecstatic. An exclamation of wonder and awe (Wow! God is Great!); mantra of ecstasy in praise of the indescribable God.